Azurite LLC

Published in the United States by Azurite LLC
ISBN 978-0-9962979-1-2

Version 1.1

This book is dedicated to Susy and Abi,
I am in awe of who you are.

CONTENTS

ACKNOWLEDGEMENTS

This book would have been so much harder, and maybe even impossible, without many people who helped in many ways.

Helen Gracie – without her cheerleading of the original idea and the help in brainstorming the outline, and reassurance that yes, the world did need another book on health, I never would have started. My daughters Abi and Susy – who shared me on weekends when I was "just finishing a couple of paragraphs, I will be right there," and who listened to me waffle on and on and on and on about health and science. Dr. Robyn Kutka, Dr Sara Wood, Dr. Lylen Ferris – three of the staff physicians at Labrix who helped me with technical questions when I needed a sounding board, and Dr. Robyn and Dr. Lylen for input and edits. My Mum, Elizabeth Rhodes, who encouraged me and listened as I repeated myself ad nauseum on particular health topics and who helped read the later editions. My Dad, David Rhodes who was the first person I dared to send chapters to for some feedback – and for being kind and thoughtful with that feedback. My sister, Alison Smith, who did a simply tremendous job on editing – both the first, serious copyediting, and then final revisions. Rusty Cunning, for the support and encouragement in the early stages, and for all the long hours of graphic design and layout and brainstorming and file conversion. Dr. Randy Rogers for reading and feedback. Robin Corrarino, Rosa Costantino, Dave Gallagher, Gitte Zuberbuheler, who read and provided feedback and edits and encouragement. Angie Daschel for some copy tweaks. Scores of doctors who share their information with curious practitioners, I am grateful for the opportunity to have learned from them. Inspiration from hundreds of integrative medicine practitioners I have met who want to bring this healing approach to their patients. Women that I have met over the last few years who were excited about the idea and wanted me to keep writing the book because they were hungry for this information and knew plenty of other women who also were. My friends, Patti, Susan, Kirsti, Steve, for your encouragement, and David – who sent me some great links to wonderful resources. Michelle Huntington who is about to help me get the word out! And to Dr. Erin Lommen, for her consistent and unwavering guidance, support, and encouragement to be everything I am.

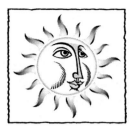

INTRODUCTION

Greetings. Thank you for picking up this book and being curious about its contents. I am a working mom who has always been interested in alternative approaches to medicine, and my work as a business woman in the medical field opened my mind to some powerful new information about health and wellness. As sales and marketing director for a healthcare organization I found myself at many conferences in the Integrative Medicine field. I listened to hundreds of lectures about how the body functions, read scores of fascinating new studies and books, and began to grasp some key pieces of information needed to understand chronic disease and options for healing. Surrounded by passionate and curious healthcare practitioners wanting to provide amazing medicine, I gradually realized that part of my work is to bring this information to their potential patients, and that is what this book is about.

According to the American Centers for Disease Control (CDC), seventy percent of American healthcare spending goes towards treatment of chronic health conditions such as heart disease, cancer and diabetes. By 2020 there will be an estimated one hundred and fifty seven million people in the US suffering with at least one form of chronic disease. The system we have in healthcare today has not been effective at finding solutions to chronic disease, and it is time for something different, something more. Forward thinking healthcare practitioners, especially those practicing Integrative Medicine, are looking for solutions that support patients on a path back to wellness and in so doing, increase positive patient outcomes for chronic disease and also help curb spending on healthcare.

The huge explosion in medical information that occurred in the twentieth century resulted in much specialization within the medical industry. Primary Care practitioners do the intake and initial tests and then patients are frequently referred to a specialist for more tests and treatment. Many times this approach is very helpful and patients definitely benefit from the specific knowledge that a specialist has. Conventional medicine does, however, tend to look at an isolated group of symptoms first, which usually results in a disease diagnosis. Often, this diagnosis is associated with a drug or drugs that can be prescribed to treat this group of symptoms, and that can be the end of the specialist's treatment strategy. While this medical approach can be life-saving for acute illness and emergency situations, when it comes to chronic problems, it may mean symptoms are suppressed and root causes never uncovered. Using the current treatment approach, people with complex problems often experience mediocre results especially over time as the body becomes used to, and sometimes resistant to, the drugs being taken. In addition, people often experience side effects from the treatment itself which leads to more illness and more drugs.

Chronic illness is often due to systemic imbalance – the result of deficiencies, toxicities, allergies, infections, immune system malfunction, and so on. This imbalance causes the body to respond with processes such as inflammation or oxidative stress, which wash over many of the 'body systems' and lead to a variety of dysfunctions. For example, conditions as diverse as heart disease, dementia and osteoporosis can all result from inflammation. A practitioner of Integrative Medicine will approach these problems by looking for the sources or 'triggers' of this inflammation and address each of those triggers. This is usually done by supplying something that is missing (e.g. nutrients) or removing things that do not belong (e.g. toxins, allergens, infections, etc.). By restoring balance, the body's natural healing mechanisms can respond.

Chronic illnesses are complex and, as mounting data shows, they need a different approach to managing care and healing. Integrative Medicine, sometimes known as Functional Medicine, looks to address the underlying causes of illness, using a systems-oriented approach and engages both patient and practitioner in a therapeutic partnership. It is an evolution in the practice of medicine that better addresses many healthcare needs of the twenty-first century.

The term Integrative Medicine refers to the blending of alternative practices with conventional medical care. There is no official list of what Integrative Medicine actually comprises, but treatments typically can include naturopathy, acupuncture, nutritional counseling, homeopathy, osteopathy, chiropractic, herbal medicine, Reiki, meditation, massage, aromatherapy, hypnosis, Ayurveda, and several other treatments not normally prescribed by conventional medicine practitioners.

By shifting the traditional disease-centered focus of medical practice to a more patient-centered approach, Integrative Medicine addresses the whole person, not just an isolated set of symptoms. Integrative Medicine practitioners spend time with their patients, listening to their histories and looking at the interactions among genetic, environmental and lifestyle factors that can influence long-term health and complex, chronic disease. In this way Integrative Medicine supports the unique expression of health and vitality for each individual.

If you are chronically tired, overweight, miserable, constantly in pain, maybe dealing with feelings of hopelessness, it is time for you to learn that there are solutions. Also know that there is no magic pill that will make it all better. It probably took years for your health to get to this point, and so it could take many months of concerted effort on your part to bring your body back to full health. You also need to be prepared to pay out of pocket for both testing and food/supplements that will help heal the "dis-ease" in your body as this kind of Functional Medicine is not always covered by health insurance plans. Whether you are up for that is up to you. Whether you are simply curious about options, or ready to take action – read on.

This book is laid out with simplicity. I am not a clinician, I make no recommendations regarding treatment approaches. The information in this book is well established basic biochemistry gathered from hundreds of peer reviewed articles and books that I have coalesced into one place. Each chapter explores different aspects of biochemistry related directly to health that will help you understand how your body works. At the end of each chapter is a summary of the key content covered. I will emphasize over and over that while you can make some of the changes on your own, your greatest success will come from working with a health care practitioner who understands the larger system of the body and has a range of tools to use related to Integrative Medicine. It is also important for you to grasp and internalize the point that medicine is an Art. Medicine uses science for the practice of the Art of medicine, that is probably why health care providers are called Practitioners. The body is so complex and the mind is so crafty at getting what it thinks it wants, that the best healthcare practitioner in the world is only going to be as successful as the patient allows. Your healthcare practitioner is your skillful guide – you will do the work.

If you are like many people nowadays, you probably cannot even remember what it feels like to be truly well, but as you start on your path of treatment with your practitioner, know that before too long, you will begin to rebuild energy and enthusiasm, regain flexibility and easy movement, and you will begin to feel like yourself again. It is my earnest, deepest, heartfelt wish that you will find something in this book that resonates with you, makes a difference, and starts you on your path back to wellness.

It takes brawn, brains and beauty to survive in this world, the information in this book is brought to you with love – to help you build the strong body, the healthy brain, the beautiful spirit, that you need to be a survivor. I invite you to turn the next page, and the next, in both this book and in your life.

Peace and abundant blessings

CHAPTER ONE

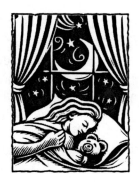

A GOOD NIGHT'S SLEEP

There are lots and lots of joys in my life, some big, most small, and right there up close to the top of the list is the time when I pull back the covers on my bed, lie down on my soft mattress and puffy pillows, and settle myself quietly into sleep. Most nights I accomplish this easily, and sleep for at least seven and a half hours before my alarm or the chink of light around the blind awakens me. Most mornings I feel refreshed, stirring awake without the need for coffee. Now that I am a morning person, it is relatively easy for me to be up like a lark and ready for the day. But if I do not get my required hours of sleep, then the morning will drag. There are mornings like this, sometimes it has been a later night, busy running around after two teenage daughters, catching up with laundry after one of my frequent work trips, restoring a façade of order to the house, or just getting a jump on the next day's meal preparation. Sometimes the night has been fraught with fear filled dreams or a night sweat or two. Sometimes my ear plugs have fallen out and the sounds of bird song or traffic will seep into my early morning sleep. Whatever the reason, if I do not get my allotted unconscious downtime, the day will bring challenges in concentration, comprehension, coordination, and communication, all of which are essential for my work day and parenting evening.

My family and close friends know that I allow very little to get in the way of my regular bedtime. By 9 pm, I am winding down. My bedtime tea is made, I switch off lights as if electricity is rationed, I am yawning repeatedly, I have finished cleaning up the kitchen, and the laptop is dark. Saying goodnight to my daughters (whom I know will be up long after me), I pull down the blackout blind, open my bedroom window to let in the cool air, insert my ear plugs, and slide under the quilt. I make a conscious effort to calm my brain down, preparing myself for sleep. I breathe deeply and, feeling my body relax, release negative energies from the day and lie still.

This has not always been the case. As a "poor sleeper" though my teenage years and through much of my early adult life, I struggled to fall sleep night after night after night. I have diaries from my high school years where I would track the times I fell asleep – 1 a.m., 2 a.m. times were common, with some nights as late as 3.30 a.m. Struggling to rise at 7.45 a.m. in time to get ready for school, there were days at a time where I barely ate breakfast and subsisted on coffee and sugar in order to lurch through the day. As for my school work, let's just leave those details inside the Pandora's box.

When I married, sleep problems continued. At the time I was a night owl, able to stay awake until midnight and beyond. My husband was the opposite, needing to be in bed with the light off by 10.30 p.m. at the latest. Reading with the light on was naturally a disruption for him and so I would take myself off to the sofa to read, and fall asleep there, stirring through the night on the uneven surface. Add two babies in two years into the mix and I lost all hope of ever getting a good night's sleep.

As I got older, not only was falling asleep difficult, but staying asleep became harder. Stresses that life brings – parenting, relationships, working, managing money, running a household, meant that my sleep cycles became even more disrupted. Ever vigilant for a sound from one of my daughters, my brain busy thinking about all the things that worried me, it could take a long time to fall asleep and then I would wake easily from anything but the deepest sleep and be on alert for upwards of thirty minutes before I fell back to sleep again. The cumulative sleep debt had an impact on my thinking, my processing, my decision making ability, my body, my mental health, my spirituality, and my nutrition decisions. I finally learned what my former husband had known all along – nothing should get in the way of a good nights' sleep, every night.

What is it that sleep gives us? What happens when we do not get enough sleep? More importantly for many, many busy people, what happens when we do not get enough sleep consistently, when we run up a cumulative sleep debt? Opinions have varied for centuries about why we need sleep, and some people do in fact appear to need very little sleep in order to function. But for most people, sleep is critical for long term physical and mental health. The best way to grasp why we need sleep is to look at what happens when we do not get sleep. There are some major body systems that start to deteriorate very, very quickly: brain functions such as concentration, decision making, emotion management, thought processing, and speech, are all affected by lack of sleep. There are physical changes such as slower response times to stimuli or when moving the head and limbs, plus lowered immunity and reduced resistance to disease. In addition, the ageing process may actually speed up with persistent lack of sleep. We know that some torture methods can include depriving prisoners of sleep. After several days of being kept awake, and often in physical discomfort, people can be driven insane as a result of the brain on sensory overload and the body riddled with pain.

Research into the purpose of sleep has been occurring for almost two centuries, however modern brain scan technology developed in the last fifteen years has provided the opportunity to learn significantly more about sleep functions, including hormone release, repair processes, memory processing and storage, and the cementing of learning.

A good night's sleep consists of cycles and different stages of sleep – the diagram below illustrates a common pattern.

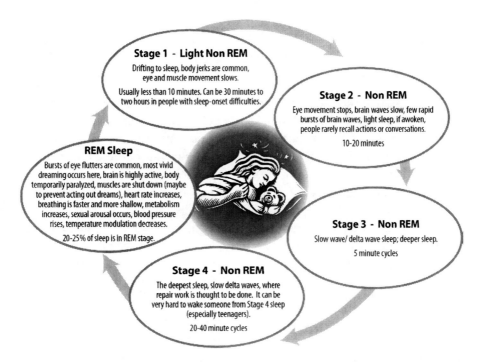

Stage 1 - Light Non REM
Drifting to sleep, body jerks are common, eye and muscle movement slows.
Usually less than 10 minutes. Can be 30 minutes to two hours in people with sleep-onset difficulties.

Stage 2 - Non REM
Eye movement stops, brain waves slow, few rapid bursts of brain waves, light sleep, if awoken, people rarely recall actions or conversations.
10-20 minutes

REM Sleep
Bursts of eye flutters are common, most vivid dreaming occurs here, brain is highly active, body temporarily paralyzed, muscles are shut down (maybe to prevent acting out dreams), heart rate increases, breathing is faster and more shallow, metabolism increases, sexual arousal occurs, blood pressure rises, temperature modulation decreases.
20-25% of sleep is in REM stage.

Stage 3 - Non REM
Slow wave/ delta wave sleep; deeper sleep.
5 minute cycles

Stage 4 - Non REM
The deepest sleep, slow delta waves, where repair work is thought to be done. It can be very hard to wake someone from Stage 4 sleep (especially teenagers).
20-40 minute cycles

We progress through stages One to Four, non REM, then REM, and then cycle back through the pattern over the entire night. It seems that the first few hours of sleep are there to satisfy the metabolic (energy managing) needs of the body, and that the later hours of sleep are to manage brain needs. It is actually common and perfectly okay to wake briefly during the night – particularly during the later stages of sleep in the transition to and from REM sleep. These transitions are short and many people do not even remember them.

How much sleep do we need?

The National Sleep Foundation recommends the following:

Age	Recommended Hours of Sleep
0-2 Months	*Ha!*
3-11 Months	14-15 Hours
1-3 Years	12-14 Hours
Preschoolers	11-13 Hours
School Age	10-11 Hours
Adults	7+ Minimum

Through thousands of years of evolution, human physiology has adapted to flow with diurnal light/dark cycles using an internal biological clock that governs the response to light and day. There is a part of the hypothalamus in the brain called the suprachiasmatic nucleus (SCN for short), which acts as the control center for diurnal rhythms. The retinas at the back of the eyes pick up messages about the amount of light or dark and send those messages to the SCN. The SCN then sends messages out to parts of the body and brain to produce hormones and neurotransmitters that control sleep, physical activity, alertness, hormone levels, body temperature, immune function, and digestive activity. In addition to the eyes, there are also light sensors in the skin, blood and bones, which all contribute to this communication process.

There are certain things that are supposed to happen in the body when it is dark and certain things that are supposed to happen when it is light. Way back in the day when the human species wandered the plains, when it was light – humans got up and went about the business of hunting and gathering. When it was dark – it was time to sleep because it wasn't

> ### { Hormone }
>
> A chemical substance produced in the body that controls and regulates the activity of certain cells or organs. Many hormones are secreted by specialized glands such as the thyroid gland. Hormones are essential for every activity of daily living, including the processes of digestion, metabolism, growth, and more.
>
> ### { Neurotransmitter }
>
> A chemical in the brain that transmits messages between neurons, or nerve cells. Changes in the levels of certain neurotransmitters, such as serotonin, norepinephrine, and dopamine have an impact on mood and function.

possible to see anything and wandering around in the dark could result in becoming a midnight snack for a predator. The discovery of fire provided a little bit more time to play with – but not much, and fires needed fuel to keep them going so there was no major demand for them as a light source, chain saws not being available at that time.

As humans moved inside caves, tents, other structures, and finally buildings, the invention of candles and oil lamps provided further light to continue activities after the sun had set. However, the diurnal cycles of light and dark still ruled. This meant that in summer – people rose when it was light at 5 a.m. and went to bed later when it got dark at 10 p.m. In winter of course, the day was significantly shorter, humans therefore developed not only diurnal patterns, but seasonal patterns as well.

Here is a really important point to note and keep in your mind at all times: the "modern" human species has been evolving gradually, incrementally, for two hundred thousand years or more. Current day humans have had artificial light accessible whenever it was needed it for less than one hundred years. Physiology and biochemistry has not had time to evolve to catch up with this artificially longer day, so when we act out of alignment with ancient physiology, there are likely to be consequences. The brain, and therefore the body, has no way to make the fast evolutionary changes asked of it by modern day perpetual light, and so cells and organs, after maybe managing to keep up for a while, will eventually begin to malfunction.

Sleep and Eating

Setting aside for now the experiences of busy modern life, of how "evolved and developed" we are as a species now, when we go back mentally to Paleolithic hunter-gatherer time in human history, things look very different. The two human primal drives as a species are to eat enough to survive and mature, and then mate to ensure survival of the species. In fact, it is the same drive in every species; these are the two primal drives sitting in the oldest parts of our brains. Everything else after that is window dressing.

In summer there is a relative abundance of food. Fruits are on the bushes, animals have produced their young, tubers grow in the ground. In winter, food resources are in shorter supply and it is often cold. Human bodies have evolved to equate light with summer and the drive to find as much food as possible to store fat ready to survive the lean times of winter. Hunting and gathering was essential for survival. People hunted and gathered and ate as much as they could to not only keep going each day, but to build up fat reserves, knowing that for four to five months of the year there could be very little food available. This wasn't a behavioral choice, it was a biologically programmed imperative. At the most fundamental of levels, Light equals "eat and put on fat or die later". This human survival instinct has been going on for hundreds of thousands of years – it is in our biochemistry, woven through us like the veins and arteries in our circulatory system.

How does the process of making fat work? The answer is found in the role of carbohydrate. The common name for carbohydrate is sugar, and the two words are used here interchangeably. When sugars are consumed, the energy is either used immediately, or is parked in the form of glycogen stores in muscle or the liver ready for when it will be needed later. Human bodies are designed to make and store fat in order to survive. Sugars are the only food that bodies can store. It does not matter if carbohydrates are refined, complex or simple, all are sugars, and sugar is what the body craves in order to make fat and increase the chances of survival.

We instantly grasp this concept when we think of bears that eat berries, prey, and the remains of summer picnics. We comprehend that bears are driven to eat as much as possible, not only for maintenance during the summer months, but to build up fat for survival during hibernation. Human biochemistry is driven by the same need to eat carbohydrate and make fat – just in case.

There is a chain of events that happens when we eat sugars:

Levels of glucose (blood sugar) have to remain within a fairly narrow band – too much glucose is just as dangerous as too little glucose. The hormone Insulin is really, really important because it directly controls what happens to glucose to ensure use and storage of fuel. Insulin has two

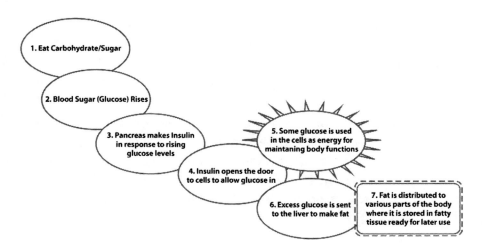

1. Eat Carbohydrate/Sugar

2. Blood Sugar (Glucose) Rises

3. Pancreas makes Insulin in response to rising glucose levels

4. Insulin opens the door to cells to allow glucose in

5. Some glucose is used in the cells as energy for maintaning body functions

6. Excess glucose is sent to the liver to make fat

7. Fat is distributed to various parts of the body where it is stored in fatty tissue ready for later use

major functions – it gives the cells access to glucose to be used in maintaining body functions, and it signals when to store excess glucose as fat. As the diagram below shows, cells have docking stations (receptors) on them for all sorts of hormones and other chemical messengers. When insulin "docks" onto the correct receptor on the cell, it acts as a key to open up the door into the cell to allow glucose to go inside to be used or stored as glycogen. If glucose levels rise above a certain threshold, it is insulin's job to shuttle excess glucose off to the liver to be converted to fat.

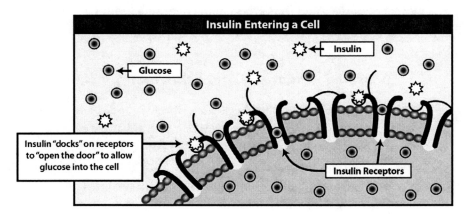

Insulin Entering a Cell

Insulin

Glucose

Insulin "docks" on receptors to "open the door" to allow glucose into the cell

Insulin Receptors

There are some additional hormones named prolactin, leptin and melatonin that play a significant role in the process of fat store accumulation. Prolactin is important not only for making milk in a lactating mother, but also for managing immune function and for controlling appetite. When prolactin levels rise, feelings of hunger are stimulated; conversely, when prolactin levels are low, there are fewer feelings of hunger. Prolactin production is regulated partly as a response to melatonin production. When melatonin levels are high, a feedback loop will lower prolactin levels. When prolactin levels drop, then there are likely to be far fewer hunger signals. Prolactin's impact on appetite works on a diurnal, or daily basis.

Leptin also manages appetite by controlling the drive to replenish fat supplies – but it works on a more seasonal basis. Leptin comes from the body's fat base and is a longer term signaling mechanism to indicate when it is time to start carbohydrate loading to build more fat supplies. If fat supplies are adequate, then leptin levels will be high. If fat supplies are low, then the corresponding lower leptin levels will signal that it is time to eat carbohydrate to rebuild fat supplies.

Diurnal Patterns of Melatonin and Appetite

Melatonin is produced at night, when it is dark. Melatonin is the hormone that sends the signal to calm down many body processes and get the brain and body ready for the nightly fast during sleep. Melatonin levels influence prolactin levels for short term management of appetite signals. As melatonin levels rise, prolactin levels start to drop. As prolactin levels drop, leptin levels will rise which decreases appetite for carbohydrate. This is why it is possible to go for several hours overnight without getting hungry as illustrated on the left hand side of the next diagram.

Seasonal Patterns of Melatonin and Appetite

In winter, a seasonal pattern occurs; when it is dark for a greater number of hours, body systems are designed to mini-hibernate, slowing all body processes and letting the body burn existing stores of fat through the winter. When days are short and nights are long, there will be much higher and consistent levels of melatonin. The higher levels of melatonin decreases prolactin, which increases leptin, which decreases appetite. Great feedback mechanisms!

In summer, when days are much longer and carbohydrate is once again available, the pattern reverses. Because days are long and nights are short, less melatonin is made and therefore more prolactin is produced. Increased prolactin lowers levels of leptin, which signals the craving for carbohydrate to start rebuilding fat supplies as shown in the middle sec-

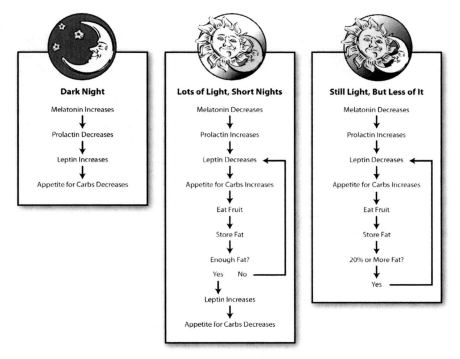

Dark Night	Lots of Light, Short Nights	Still Light, But Less of It
Melatonin Increases	Melatonin Decreases	Melatonin Decreases
↓	↓	↓
Prolactin Decreases	Prolactin Increases	Prolactin Increases
↓	↓	↓
Leptin Increases	Leptin Decreases ←	Leptin Decreases ←
↓	↓	↓
Appetite for Carbs Decreases	Appetite for Carbs Increases	Appetite for Carbs Increases
	↓	↓
	Eat Fruit	Eat Fruit
	↓	↓
	Store Fat	Store Fat
	↓	↓
	Enough Fat?	20% or More Fat?
	Yes No	↓
	↓	Yes
	Leptin Increases	
	↓	
	Appetite for Carbs Decreases	

tion of the diagram. In summer, when fruits are on the trees and bushes and roots are plentiful, there is plenty of time to harvest and eat, and the chemical messages support that.

Now, there is an interesting quirk to the seasonal system in late summer. When nights begin to shorten again, a different feedback mechanism begins. The brain senses the shortening days and focuses on continuing to build fat supplies for the winter. As the right hand side of the diagram shows, as fat is stored, if fat supplies are greater than twenty pounds or so, this can actually completely stop production of leptin. Remember that elevated leptin levels reduce appetite. With no leptin and therefore nothing suppressing the appetite for carbohydrate, the brain wants carbs, carbs, carbs, to build up body fat for the winter.

This system worked well back in cave dwelling days when there truly was a dark winter with limited carbohydrate available. However, fast forward to modern day: while the biochemistry is still the same, the amount of light and the regular supply of carbohydrate is vastly different. Body systems are working the same way they have always done, but now there is light whenever it is needed, and carbohydrate is there sitting in the fridge, the grocery store and the coffee shop; we can even have it delivered in under thirty minutes in the form of pizza.

We are no longer at the mercy of the elements and a seasonal clock, today it takes lifestyle decisions made consciously to effect control of this biochemical drive. Overcoming the chemical messages coming from the body is a challenge, and that is why education and information is important. Insulin production is controlled by what the brain chooses to eat, but what the brain craves to eat is controlled by the brain's perceived seasonal variations in light and current stress levels. The pattern of continuing to eat carbohydrate, to lay in supplies of fat for the (not happening) winter famine, can contribute to persistent weight gain and, eventually, to obesity. In modern day winter, with no feedback mechanism to suppress appetite, the body continues to crave carbohydrate. From a diurnal point of view, the longer we stay awake with the lights on, the more we will likely stimulate appetite.

By heading to bed in good time, by darkening the room completely and allowing plenty of time for melatonin to be produced, we increase the chance of not eating the foods that make us store fat. Remember that the SCN senses light through the retinas, skin, blood and bones. Even though eyes may be closed, attempting to sleep in a room with lights on, skin (including eyelids), will sense that light. As long as the SCN receives the message that there is light, it will slow or stop the production of melatonin. An ideal sleeping room should be completely dark to help achieve maximum melatonin production.

Sleep and Immunity

Another vital role of sleep is in maintaining and bolstering immunity. The immune system is composed of the gut (stomach, intestines etc), lymphatic system, brain, glands, and skin, and all these elements communicate in real time with each other. At first glance it might seem surprising that at least seventy percent of the immune system is located in the gut, but because a really high proportion of toxins enter the body through the mouth, it is quite natural that this should be the first line of defense. There are billions of bacteria in the gut, most with important jobs in defense and immune function, hence a balance between gut bacteria is essential for optimal health. Too many of the wrong bacteria is as risky as too few bacteria, and the body has therefore evolved a fabulous mechanism for managing bacteria levels – sleep. Melatonin and prolactin promote white cells, T cells, and killer cells, all of which are important in managing both levels of bacteria in the gut, and in mounting an important defense against disease throughout the body. No sleep, or inadequate sleep, means poor bacteria management, which contributes to an impaired immune system.

An additional benefit that sleep brings to management of gut bacteria is the change in body temperature that happens during sleep. Warm body temperatures mean that bacteria can flourish, so there is a control mechanism to lower body temperature during sleep and thus kill off some harmful bacteria. It is actually melatonin that lowers body temperature, and the purpose of lower temperatures is to slow metabolic processes and let the body fast and "not starve" overnight. Melatonin will also set the timer on ovarian and testicular function, gets the immune system ready for ramp up for the next day, and is a powerful antioxidant that helps control immunity during sleep.

Heart Health

The total hours of sleep also have a profound impact on heart health. As appetite for carbohydrate increases and as carbohydrate is consumed in response, a number of things happen. First, there is an increase of stored fat in several areas of the body. Second, carbohydrate molecules contain a high proportion of water so there is an increase in water retention which changes blood pressure. Third, insulin production increases in order to manage blood sugar, which, in turn causes cholesterol to rise.

We are designed to have seasonal metabolism, just like we are designed to have seasonal brains. Winter is supposed to be the time we use up those fatty acids accumulated in summer. If those fatty acids are not used up, they will likely accumulate in the arteries. Arteries are lined with a thin layer of endothelial cells called the endothelium that is in direct contact with blood flow. The endothelial cells job is to try to ensure that blood pressure is as smooth and regular as possible. Endothelial cells also help control how fatty acids are metabolized by the body. Unfortunately, chronic stress and increases in blood pressure can kill the endothelial cells. Even ten to fifteen pounds of extra weight from a high carbohydrate diet is enough to

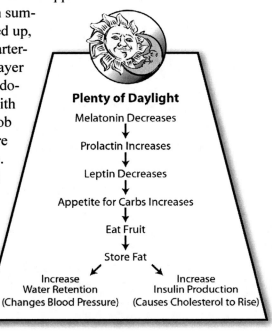

Plenty of Daylight

Melatonin Decreases
↓
Prolactin Increases
↓
Leptin Decreases
↓
Appetite for Carbs Increases
↓
Eat Fruit
↓
Store Fat
↙   ↘
Increase   Increase
Water Retention   Insulin Production
(Changes Blood Pressure) (Causes Cholesterol to Rise)

raise blood pressure and change heart health. There is a bacterium called Endotoxin LPS which is released in the gut and this can also damage the endothelial cells if the levels of endotoxin LPS rise too high. Endotoxin LPS is "killed off" by a drop in body temperature; which gives another reason to ensure adequate sleep, to allow body temperature to drop, and the levels of Endotoxin LPS to reduce and protect your heart.

Lack of sleep impacts cortisol levels. Cortisol is a steroid hormone produced in the adrenal gland. It is the "fight or flight" hormone, the chemical messenger that tracks the immediate environment and is alert for anything that might be dangerous. There is much more information about cortisol in the Chapters on Hormones and Stress, however for now, know that when cortisol levels are elevated then there may be risk to the endothelial cells. A balanced amount of cortisol is good, it helps the endothelial cells work well, but consistently high levels of cortisol can cause the endothelial cells to die off. Making sure that you prepare the body for rest and sleep goes a long way to helping bring down cortisol levels at the end of the day.

If we are supposed to spend at least seven hours in the complete dark each day, and up to thirteen hours at the depths of winter, it is clear that in today's world there is a major disconnect between what the body has evolved to need and what it actually gets. The invention of the light bulb was wonderful in many ways, it allowed exponential expansion of technical capacity because we could work longer and do so many more functions with lights on than with lights off. However, in the last forty years or so, in many developed countries, life styles and sleeping patterns have adjusted so significantly that many people no longer achieve even the barest minimum of sleep.

There are a number of factors that can cause inadequate sleep beyond simply staying up too late, burning the candle at both ends, or sleeping with the lights or the TV on. There are many medical disorders that can affect the amount of sleep we get and entire books have been written on the subject, so here is a quick review of the most common sleep disorders.

Obstructive Sleep Apnea (OSA)

If you sleep next to some who snores loudly, gasps for air, experiences lapses in breathing and jerks suddenly at repeated times during the night – you may be sleeping next to someone with OSA. If your bed partner is the one poking and growling at you for snoring and jerking all night, it may be you have sleep apnea. Sleep apnea, although sounding undramatic, has quite serious implications for long term health from a number of perspectives.

During sleep the soft tissues of the back of the mouth and throat will relax and can hang down, thus blocking the windpipe. If the airway is completely blocked then air cannot flow down into and out of the lungs. Breathing may stop for as long as a minute and then levels of oxygen in the blood begin to drop. This is not good! The body is definitely going to jerk to attention in this situation. In addition to the stress that OSA can put on heart and lungs, OSA interferes significantly with restful sleep, and the resulting fatigue reduces the capacity to concentrate, raises the chance of depression, increases the risk of heart disease, decreases over-all functioning capability and can have a negative impact on important partner relationships.

Apnea events are more likely to occur during light non-REM and REM sleep and less so in deep non-REM sleep. While a partner or family member woken by the sound of snoring (again!) may alert the sleeper to the possibility of sleep apnea, diagnosis will usually require a sleep study. The sleep study measures electrical activity in the brain and muscles, eye movement, heart patterns, air flow and how hard the chest is working, how open is the airway to the lungs. A practitioner will interpret the results, diagnose any sleep issues, and develop a treatment plan.

Risk factors for OSA include excess body weight especially obesity, a short, thick neck with a circumference greater than seventeen and a half inches, large tongue, receding jaw-line, menopause, smoking, asthma, epilepsy, enlarged tonsils and adenoids, a previous broken nose. Things that can make OSA worse are drinking alcohol before bedtime, weight gain and rhinitis (post nasal drip).

Insomnia

Insomnia can be defined as having repeated difficulty in falling asleep and/or staying asleep, waking up too early, and/or feeling unrefreshed or unrested the following day. Insomnia affects over fifty percent of American adults at some point in their lives, and a research study in the UK estimated that thirty seven percent of adults experience insomnia. Australians are the world's longest sleepers, with seventy three percent catching eight hours or more a night, compared with forty nine percent globally. Source: An AC Nielson poll.

Insomnia affects energy level, mood, and the immune system. It can cause feelings of sleepiness or fatigue during the day and result in reduced ability to focus on tasks. Fatigue leads to diminished mental alertness and concentration. Poor sleepers have been found to receive fewer promotions, to show poor productivity, and to have increased absent-mindedness. Lack of sleep is linked to accidents on the road and on the job, and sleep deprivation can impact the brain's performance in the same way that alcohol can.

Insomniacs can be divided into three main groups:

- Insomnia driven by the sleep environment. In this category a person may have trouble falling asleep due to too much noise, too much light, or body jerks or other movement from a bed partner.
- Those who prepare for bed with good sleep hygiene, but who still cannot fall asleep, ending up tossing and turning and watching the dark.
- People who have a lot to do and not enough time to do it in, who actively decide to stay awake to complete tasks e.g. work, homework, emails, housework, volunteer work, playing games.

Stress can have a significant impact on the capacity to fall asleep. Cortisol was mentioned earlier in the chapter and it will come up more later, but it is important to reiterate that if a person is under stress, it is likely that the adrenal glands will be producing more cortisol in response to that stress. When cortisol levels are high, it is very difficult to go to sleep because the brain and body are "on alert". The level of stress has a significant impact on the amount of sleep disruption. Events such as divorce, death in the family, trauma, job loss are all situations that can cause extreme stress and impact sleep significantly. Other activities and circumstances can contribute to disruption of sleep patterns including changes in work or school routine, injury, jet lag, major organ disease, persistent pain, some medications, hormone imbalances, and of course, consumption of too much caffeine – including that in chocolate! (Sorry).

Insomnia is also often linked to depression and anxiety, poor gut health or some sort of sleep disorder. It is important to get help for insomnia because once you find yourself in a slept debt situation you are caught in a feedback loop of inadequate sleep causing reduced functioning, reduced healing, reduced capacity to cope, and this can lead to even more problems falling asleep. Know that insomnia can be a disorder in its own right, but often it is a symptom of some other disease or condition, so it is really important to find a practitioner who can help you get to the root cause of sleep issues.

Neurotransmitter Imbalances

Neurotransmitters are chemicals in the brain that transmit messages between neurons, or nerve cells. Some neurotransmitters are excitatory and stimulate activity in the brain, and others are inhibitory and calm brain activity. There are two important inhibitory neurotransmitters called Serotonin and GABA. Well known excitatory neurotransmitters are Dopamine, Norepinephrine, Epinephrine, and Glutamate. Having an imbalance between excitatory and inhibitory neurotransmitter levels can significantly impact the ability to fall asleep and stay asleep. If someone has persistent sleep issues, a practitioner may want to test neurotransmitter levels with a simple urine sample. This test will provide a snapshot view of the general levels of neurotransmitters being spilled into urine, and, when matched with symptoms reported, gives the practitioner more information on where to start with a treatment plan. When stress levels are high, the two neurotransmitters norepinephrine and epinephrine are likely to be high. When these excitatory neurotransmitters are firing in the brain, it can be very hard to get to sleep.

Circadian Rhythm Disorders (CRD)

People with CRDs have rhythms that do not match the usual diurnal patterns governed by light and dark. The people most affected by this are shift workers, those who travel across time zones frequently, people with internal time clocks that run too long or too short, or people who are blind. The SCN responds to the amount of light available and directs activity in the body in response to that; regulating hormones and neurotransmitters to wake up when it is light, and induce sleep when it is dark. People with circadian rhythm sleep disorders are unable to sleep and wake at the times required for normal work, school, and social needs.

Delayed Sleep Phase Disorder (DSPD) is the most common type of CRD and is defined as a chronic disorder of the timing of sleep, peak period of alertness, the core body temperature rhythm, hormonal and other daily rhythms, compared to the general population and relative to society's requirements. People with DSPD are generally able to get enough sleep if allowed to sleep and wake at the times dictated by their body clocks. Unless they have another sleep disorder, their sleep is usually of normal quality. Parents of adolescents may see this pattern appear in their teenagers who can be awake for a couple of hours after most people have gone to sleep. Left to sleep on the weekends, teenagers and young adult often sleep long and deep to catch up.

The problem with DSPD comes when it is necessary to be up early and out of the house ready to get to school or work five days a week. The accumulated sleep debt brings the problems already described, including keeping up good grades at school or performing well at work. Caffeine is a convenient crutch to put the body on alert and keep it awake, but the overuse of such stimulants can make it even harder to get to sleep at the end of the day.

In most cases, it is not known what causes the abnormality in the biological clocks of some with DSPS (it does tend to run in families so it's probably a genetic variant), but there are some actions that can help with adjusting and maintaining rhythms. Light therapy in the morning can help move the body clock a little earlier, as can keeping dim lighting in the house before bedtime. Melatonin is an over the counter supplement that can be used in small doses to help signal that it is time for sleep, but always ask a practitioner for guidance in the use of supplements because too much can cause side effects including disrupted sleep later in the sleep cycle.

Maintaining a strict schedule and good sleep hygiene are essential tricks in maintaining any good effects of treatment. With treatment, some people with mild DSPS may sleep and function well with an early sleep schedule. A big difficulty of treating DSPS is in maintaining an earlier schedule after it has been established. Inevitable events of normal life, such as staying up late for a celebration or to work on homework, or having to stay in bed with an illness, tend to reset the sleeping schedule to its natural later times.

Shift Work

Shift-lag is a new term appearing in our vocabulary. As the global marketplace "advances," more and more employees are needed to work unconventional shifts that do not match the natural diurnal rhythm. Nearly twenty percent of employees in industrialized countries are employed in shift work, which requires them to drastically change their sleep habits weekly or even daily. Electric light has made it possible to work around the clock, and many modern day industrial and service functions cannot operate successfully anymore without twenty-four-seven activity. Nowhere are the effects of lifestyle on sleep more evident than in shift work disorder, also called shift work change and shift lag. Shift work creates irregular sleep times, poor daytime sleep environments, plus job and family pressures. All the problems of concentration, decision making, emotion management, thought processing and speech referred to earlier, are compounded by shift work. The structural tips below on Sleep Hygiene are critical resources for shift workers who often complete their day just as the rest of the world is getting started.

Restless Legs Syndrome (RLS)

Hard to pin down and define, RLS is experienced in many different ways, and occurs on a spectrum of intensity. It is defined as the irresistible urge to move the legs in some way, and is accompanied by feelings of aching, tingling, vibrations running through the limbs, and also creeping and crawling sensations deep inside the muscles or bones. The urge can occur as often as every five seconds or as much as ten to fifteen minute intervals. Where it causes a problem is when it disrupts sleep either when getting ready to fall asleep or to the point of waking a person during sleep. RLS can also have a significant impact on a bed partner.

The most commonly associated medical condition linked to RLS is iron deficiency but it can also be related to a whole host of conditions including varicose veins, folate deficiency, magnesium deficiency, low dopamine levels, fibromyalgia, sleep apnea, kidney disease, diabetes, thyroid disease, Parkinson's disease, and some autoimmune diseases. In addition, some medications are known to cause RLS while caffeine, tobacco and nicotine can trigger RLS, or make it worse. Like other sleep disorders, the impact is poor sleep and a gradually accumulating sleep debt, so anyone experiencing RLS should discuss this with a practitioner.

Other sleep disorders that can significantly reduce the amount of sleep include: excessive daytime sleepiness (hypersomnia), sleep walking, night terrors, sleep related binge eating, and sleep talking. All can have the same impact – reduced sleep and reduced functioning.

Sleep Hygiene Checklist

Restful sleep improves health by allowing the body to repair itself at the cellular level. Rituals and routines keep the body in rhythm. The suggestions below can support development of healthy sleep habits.

Structural Tips

- First – rename the bedroom (if only mentally) as the sleeproom. Make the mental adjustment to think of the sleeproom as an oasis, a safe place.

- Try to use the bedroom only for sleep (and intimacy). Use other areas of the house for working and for TV watching, reading, game playing and computer use.
- Avoid writing, working, eating, watching TV, using a lap top, talking on the phone, or playing cards while in bed.
- Make the bedroom quiet and a little bit cool, but make sure there are enough blankets and covers to stay warm as body temperature drops.
- Use blackout shades to keep out as much light as possible.
- Make sure the bed is comfortable. A queen sized bed should be large enough for two peaceful sleepers; a king size may be better if one person is restless, or two separate beds is another option.

Daily actions to prepare for sleep

- Wake up at the same approximate time each morning; even on weekends and holidays and keep to a regular schedule.
- Avoid taking naps if possible, especially after 3 p.m.
- Avoid any caffeine after lunch.
- Avoid any alcohol within four to six hours of bedtime.
- Avoid cigarettes or any other source of nicotine before bedtime.
- Try to exercise often but avoid any strenuous exercise within four hours of bedtime.
- We sweat overnight, so air the bedding out each morning so it is dry for the evening.

Evening preparation

- Begin turning lights off as it gets closer to bedtime - using incandescent light bulbs can cause disruptions in a person's sleeping cycle. Continuous exposure to incandescent light bulbs can cause a person to feel that their days are longer.
- Close down the computer, finish games, and turn off the TV about thirty minutes before bedtime to allow the brain to calm down from the stimulus of action and color and sound.
- Begin rituals that help relaxation each night before bed. This can include activities such as a warm bath, a light snack or a few minutes of reading.

- Avoid going to bed unless sleepy. If not sleepy at bedtime, then do something else to relax the body and distract the mind.
- Avoid going to bed hungry, but also avoid eating a big meal near bedtime. A few grams of protein before bed can be helpful.
- Avoid sleeping pills. If sleeping aids are used regularly, even over the counter, consult a practitioner.
- Focus on a clear mind: keep a bedside journal to jot things down that cause worry and anxiety.
- Use ear plugs to dull sound and reduce the number of sounds that may startle you – this is particularly important if experiencing stress.
- If not asleep after twenty minutes, get out of bed and find something else to do that is relaxing. Keep the bed for sleeping.

Sleep Diary

In the Appendix is a sleep diary. If you have trouble sleeping – either or both of falling asleep or staying asleep, complete the diary for a month. Add notes about what was going on at the time to round out the data. Your practitioner will be able to use this information to work with you on a treatment plan.

Conclusion

This chapter explores the natural biochemical rhythms influencing sleep which have developed over thousands years of human evolution. There is an explanation why sleep is important for brain function and for metabolic function. There is a review of a few of the common sleep disorders that occur in modern day society and then a list of some of the steps you can start taking to help yourself move towards better sleep and more sleep. Not enough sleep can make you tired, miserable, incompetent, overweight, dangerous (e.g. in charge of a car/plane/train/bus), and increase your risk of developing serious health issues as you get older. If you have persistent problems with sleeping, it is really important that you talk with your practitioner. Sleep is nature's way of making life a whole lot better. When we rest the body and the brain on a consistent basis, then anything can become possible.

"The amount of sleep required by the average person is five minutes more"

Wilson Mizener

"People who say they sleep like a baby usually don't have one"

Leo J. Burke

Chapter One Summary – Sleep

- Review of the biological imperatives of adequate sleep
- Overview of the stages of sleep
- How the brain responds to light and dark cycles
- How weight can change in response to light and dark cycles
- The role of melatonin in sleep and appetite
- Sleep issues including sleep apnea, insomnia, circadian rhythm disorder, shift work, restless leg syndrome
- Tips for good sleep hygiene

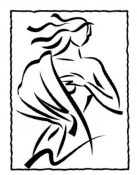

HORMONES

Hormones, *ah hormones* – there are very few women who have not found themselves at the mercy of their hormones at some point in their lives. We only have to recall the chaos of puberty, PMS, hot flashes or night sweats, to know that sometimes it doesn't matter how hard we try, how much we think we are in control as a developed species – hormonal biochemistry always has a strong set of trump cards. Few other medical topics elicit such a wide range of responses and are so frequently discussed, as hormones. This chapter aims to explain some basic biochemistry that will be relevant to your understanding of hormone function and how hormones impact you. The body has over thirty known hormones, however in this chapter the focus is on the following steroid hormones - the sex hormones Estradiol, Estriol, Estrone, Progesterone, Testosterone; and the adrenal hormones Cortisol and DHEA (Dihydroepiandosterone).

Hormones are the chemical messengers that start and stop different functions throughout the body. Hormones are made in the endocrine glands which together form what is called the endocrine system. Although we rarely think about the endocrine system, it influences almost every cell, organ, and function of the body. The endocrine system is vital in regulating mood, growth and development, tissue function, metabolism, sexual function and reproductive processes, resistance to disease, and response to stress.

When the right signals are received, hormones are released from the endocrine glands into the blood stream for delivery to other parts of the body, often far from the gland itself. However, any given hormone usually affects only a limited number of cells, known as "target cells".

A target cell responds to a hormone because it has "receptors" for that hormone. Hormones, like all molecules, have a specific molecular shape, and thus will fit into certain receptors but not others, as illustrated by the diagram below.

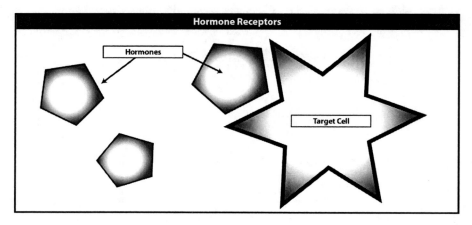

Think about bicycle messengers in cities. They are responsible for taking packages of "something" from one place to another. The package could be documents to another business, a supply of parts for a manufacturer, or take-out to a hungry tummy, but whatever the package is, it is sent from one place to be used in another. Businesses and organizations rely on the messenger system as much as the customer on the other end. A legal firm can send out a stack of documents to a business to complete the purchase of a building. If those documents don't arrive, the building purchase can't happen. Similarly, the glands in the endocrine system send out all sorts of hormones to cell receptors throughout the body. As long as the right messages are arriving at the right time in the right amount – all is good.

The diagram on the next page shows the location of the endocrine glands. Pituitary gland, Thyroid gland, Adrenal glands, Gonads (ovaries in women and testes in men), Islets (Islands) of Langerhans of the Pancreas.

How The Hormone System Functions

The body needs the following elements for the hormone system to work well:

1. Healthy endocrine glands that work correctly to make hormones,

2. A properly functioning blood supply to move hormones through the body to their target points,

3. Receptor sites on the target cells for the hormones to do their work,

4. A feedback system for controlling how and when hormones are produced and used.

Disruption to any part of the system can cause problems that may require medical intervention.

There are a group of hormones that cause other hormones to start production –these are called "releasing hormones" because their presence tells the body to release other hormones. For example, Corticotropin-Releasing Hormone causes the body to secrete cortisol. A group of proteins called Binding Globulins play a big role in the efficiency of the hormone message. These globulins will bind (stick to) hormones and stop them working as they are supposed to. An important example is Sex Hormone Binding Globulin, which will stick to circulating estrogen and testosterone hormones among others and so prevent them from entering the cell. This is important to know because a bound hormone simply cannot enter the receptor site on the target cell - it is like trying to unlock your car door with a key that has a big glob of chewing gum on it. The key will just not fit in the lock.

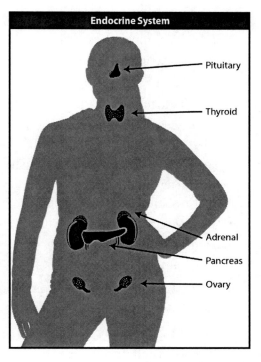

Endocrine System

Pituitary

Thyroid

Adrenal

Pancreas

Ovary

Hormone production is almost always regulated by a delicate set of feedback relationships, or "feedback loops." Most (but not all) hormone secretion is governed by "negative" feedback loops, wherein the amount of a hormone in a system regulates its own concentration. When the concentration of a hormone rises above desired levels, a series of steps happen to stop production of that hormone so the concentration will drop. The opposite happens also, when the level is too low, the body will increase concentration of that particular hormone.

Progesterone

Progesterone is really important and has lots of functions in the body, the main functions being:

- Promotes normal sleep patterns
- Calms the brain
- Reduces cholesterol
- Inhibits coronary vasospasm
- Protects against coronary hyper-reactivity
- Is a diuretic
- Helps glucose utilization and improves insulin resistance
- Enhances thyroid hormone activity by decreasing the protein Thyroid Binding Globulin
- Improves estrogen receptor sensitivity
- Balances out the effects of estrogen in the breasts, brain, and uterine lining
- Increases scalp hair
- Helps to burn fat for energy
- Is an anti-depressant
- Promotes osteoblasts (the foundation for building bone)
- Stabilizes and induces secretory endometrial changes
- Is essential for maintaining pregnancy
- Promotes cell differentiation
- Promotes normal cell death (apoptosis)

During pregnancy the developing fetus is bathed in progesterone. It is a natural hormone that helps to maintain the integrity of the uterine lining and hence helps maintain the pregnancy.

{ Progestins Are Not Progesterone }

Progestins are synthetic compounds which have a different molecular structure to the hormone progesterone. Synthetic progestins are found in birth control pills and synthetic hormone replacement medications. Progestins do not have the same effects as natural progesterone and have some negative side effects.

In women, progesterone is produced by the ovaries throughout the monthly cycle, with a large surge in the amount of progesterone during the second half of the cycle (the luteal phase). After ovulation, progesterone is released from the corpus luteum, (the sac that surrounds the egg prior to ovulation) when the egg is released from the ovary. A woman has to ovulate to produce the surge of progesterone in the second half of her cycle. Progesterone is also produced in very small amounts by the adrenal gland. Men produce progesterone in the adrenal gland.

Estrogen

There are three types of estrogen in the female body: Estrone, Estradiol, and Estriol.

Estrone is considered a weaker form of estrogen. It is typically produced by special belly fat cells, and is the major estrogen found in naturally-post menopausal women who are not using any form of synthetic hormone replacement. It is not directly active in tissues, but can be readily converted by most women to estradiol for actual use. Estrone is known to be a carcinogen as well as to cause breast tenderness or pain, nausea, headache, hypertension, and leg cramps.

Estradiol is by far the most potent of the estrogens and one that is monitored through testing most often. Estrogen has over four hundred functions, the main ones are listed here:

- Aids development of sex characteristics (women: ovaries/breasts, men: prostate)
- Stores fat
- Decreases thyroid function by increasing Thyroid Binding Globulin
- Stimulates GABA receptors in the brain
- Stimulates growth of endometrial tissue
- Stimulates development of follicle ready for ovulation
- Stimulates growth of breast tissue
- Supports healthy vaginal tissue
- Maintains collagen in skin and connective tissue
- Aids in synthesis of neurotransmitters
- Increases Serotonin
- Aids in glucose transport across the blood-brain barrier

- Sensitizes neurons to nerve growth factor
- Lowers Fibrinogen
- Inhibits vasoconstriction
- Decreases Low Density Lipoprotein ("bad" cholesterol) and Increases High Density Lipoprotein ("good" cholesterol)
- Inhibits osteoclasts (cells that reabsorb bone)
- Improves insulin sensitivity
- And much more

Estriol is a metabolic waste product of estradiol metabolism that can still have some effects on a limited number of estrogen receptors. Estriol levels are high during pregnancy as it is produced by the placenta. It is formed in the liver and is eight percent as potent as estradiol and fourteen percent as potent as estrone. Once estriol is bound to an estrogen receptor, it blocks the stronger estradiol from acting there. Thus it is considered to be a protective hormone. There is also some evidence that, because it is so weak and blocks the stronger forms of estrogen, estriol could potentially be considered to have "anti-cancer" action. More research may be needed to confirm this.

Xenoestrogens

Xenoestrogens are artificial chemicals that, due to their chemical structure, act like estrogens in the human body. They are now found in many places in the environment, for example:

- Commercially raised meat and poultry can be loaded with estrone – many animals are given hormones to help retain fluid and store fat before slaughtering
- High fat dairy products contain estrogens
- Some pesticides have similar molecular structure to estrogens
- Plastics
- Cosmetics
- Drinking water may also contain estrogens. Run off from fields where pesticides are used can gradually increase the levels of estrogen in ground water and there have also been examples of estrogen levels in river water being elevated to the point that fish

become predominantly female. The suggested reason for the increase in estrogen levels is the high use of HRT among women contributes to more estrogens washed through water treatment plants and released into rivers.

DHEA – Dihydroepiandosterone

DHEA is the most abundant hormone in the body and is produced primarily in the adrenal gland and in the brain. It exists in two forms – free DHEA and sulfated DHEA (DHEAS). DHEA is the biologically active form of the hormone, and is the only form which can be converted into the hormones testosterone, androstendione, estrone, and estradiol. Only DHEA (not DHEAS) is protective of the brain. In addition to being the base hormone for making other hormones, DHEA has an important role in the stress response. DHEA has been shown to elevate mood, calm emotions, and increase alertness – all essential qualities for responding well to stressful situations.

The main functions of DHEA are:

- Stress response management
- Important for libido and arousal
- Improves sense of motivation and well being
- Improves immune function
- Improves REM sleep function
- Improves memory function

DHEA levels in the body begin to decrease after age thirty, and are reported to be low in some people with anorexia, end-stage kidney disease, type two diabetes (non-insulin dependent diabetes), AIDS, adrenal insufficiency, and in the critically ill. DHEA levels may also be reduced by a number of drugs, including insulin, opiates, and danazol. DHEA can be converted to estradiol and to testosterone and, if levels of testosterone rise too far, it is possible to end up with side effects such as thinning hair, acne, and increased facial hair. Although DHEA is available over the counter, these products maybe stronger than is needed, so it is really important to work with a practitioner to check all your hormone levels using saliva testing and then your practitioner can help find the right balance of hormone support that works for your body.

Testosterone

Testosterone is the principal male sex hormone and, as an anabolic hormone, is responsible for building up muscle and bone. We see the effect of testosterone in men much more than women (aka, larger bones and stronger muscles, facial hair etc) but testosterone is actually very important to women too. Men make testosterone primarily in the testes and women make testosterone in the ovaries; small amounts can also be made in the adrenal gland if the adrenal gland is healthy. Testosterone can also be made through conversion of DHEA. The main functions of testosterone include:

- Improves brain function by assisting in the synthesis of neurotransmitters
- Improves sleep
- Improves sense of well-being and vitality
- Essential for libido, arousal, and orgasm
- Improves bone density
- Is anabolic and so helps to burn fat
- Testosterone can be converted to estradiol

Men usually have about ten times the level of testosterone that women do, however women are usually more sensitive to the impact of testosterone in the body, particularly in terms of sexual development. Puberty, and the onset of menstruation in girls, is triggered by a rise in production of testosterone and DHEA in the adrenal glands (known as adrenarche). In women, testosterone levels fluctuate throughout the menstrual cycle, rising just before ovulation, creating a surge in libido.

Testosterone is very important for increasing a woman's sensitivity to stimulation of the external genitals, for general libido, and for intensity in sexual satisfaction. Loss of interest in sex or in any form of sexual intimacy, and/or loss of the capacity to achieve orgasm, are commonly experienced by women who have lowered levels of testosterone. For some women, this can be a relief, but for others, the loss of intimacy and sexual connection with a loved spouse or partner can bring sadness, anxiety, and feelings of despair at losing something that was such fun and brought such pleasure.

The relationship between Estradiol and Progesterone

The interaction between the various hormones is complex. Progesterone is the natural balance to estradiol. Part of supporting a comfortable passage through perimenopause and menopause is ensuring that the balance between estradiol and progesterone is optimal. To understand what is changing, let us take a look at the usual monthly cycle.

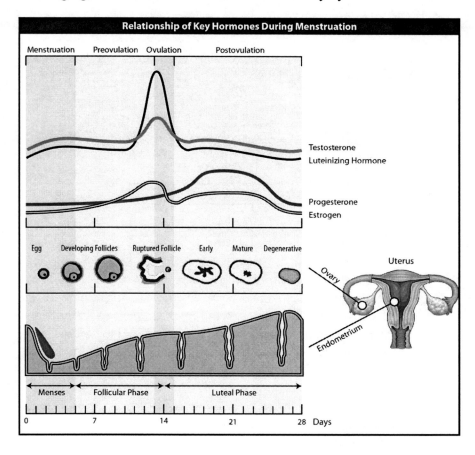

Young woman with regular cycles

The two diagrams illustrate the stages in the usual twenty eight day cycle a woman experiences. You can read through the narrative in the second diagram on the next page.

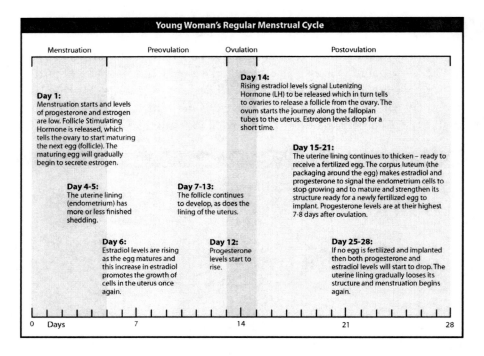

Young Woman's Regular Menstrual Cycle

| Menstruation | Preovulation | Ovulation | Postovulation |

Day 1:
Menstruation starts and levels of progesterone and estrogen are low. Follicle Stimulating Hormone is released, which tells the ovary to start maturing the next egg (follicle). The maturing egg will gradually begin to secrete estrogen.

Day 14:
Rising estradiol levels signal Lutenizing Hormone (LH) to be released which in turn tells to ovaries to release a follicle from the ovary. The ovum starts the journey along the fallopian tubes to the uterus. Estrogen levels drop for a short time.

Day 4-5:
The uterine lining (endometrium) has more or less finished shedding.

Day 7-13:
The follicle continues to develop, as does the lining of the uterus.

Day 15-21:
The uterine lining continues to thicken – ready to receive a fertilized egg. The corpus luteum (the packaging around the egg) makes estradiol and progesterone to signal the endometrium cells to stop growing and to mature and strengthen its structure ready for a newly fertilized egg to implant. Progesterone levels are at their highest 7-8 days after ovulation.

Day 6:
Estradiol levels are rising as the egg matures and this increase in estradiol promotes the growth of cells in the uterus once again.

Day 12:
Progesterone levels start to rise.

Day 25-28:
If no egg is fertilized and implanted then both progesterone and estradiol levels will start to drop. The uterine lining gradually looses its structure and menstruation begins again.

| 0 Days | 7 | 14 | 21 | 28 |

Woman hoping to conceive

An adequate amount of progesterone is crucial to a woman who is trying to become pregnant. This is because progesterone prepares the uterine wall for implantation of the fertilized egg. The luteal phase is the latter half of the menstrual cycle during which the corpus luteum produces progesterone to maintain the endometrial lining of the uterus in the hope of a fertilized egg. The length of the luteal phase should ideally be at least ten days. A defective luteal phase occurs when the length of time during which progesterone is produced (i.e. between ovulation and menstruation beginning) is insufficient to allow a fertilized egg to implant because the lining has already begun to disintegrate. Insufficient levels of progesterone, or if it is produced for too short a time, may mean the egg cannot survive inside the uterine lining. This is known as a defective or inadequate luteal phase, or luteal phase defect.

Pregnancy, with repeated miscarriage within six to eight weeks.

Progesterone is needed to facilitate implantation and to prevent rejection of the developing embryo. If a woman experiences several miscarriages within the first few weeks of the pregnancy, this may be due to luteal phase failure, where there is insufficient progesterone to support the pregnancy. Supplementing with progesterone is a safe and effective way to increase the chances of a viable pregnancy. Working with a practitioner who understands the role of natural progesterone (rather than progestins) could be a helpful step.

Changes to this pattern during perimenopause

We know what the regular monthly cycle should be, and we also know that things change for women as they move through their late thirties and into their forties. This period of time in a woman's life is known as perimenopause – the time before menopause. As a woman gets older, the cells that are to mature into eggs will age also. The remaining eggs have more difficulty maturing to a developmental stage ready for ovulation. As a result, pregnancy can be more difficult, birth defects are more frequent, menstrual cycles can be irregular, fibroids can appear and grow, the risk of breast cancer increases, bone loss begins, weight can increase and for some women it can become increasingly difficult to cope with the normal demands of life.

In terms of the monthly cycle – look again at the diagram illustrating the monthly cycle. If, instead of release of the follicle from the ovary, there is no ovulation, several things can happen. First, although there is some progesterone made from the adrenal gland and the ovary, if there is no follicle released, there will be no corpus luteum (the sac around the follicle), and if there is no corpus luteum there will be no surge of progesterone in the second half (luteal phase) of the cycle. Without that surge of progesterone, the uterine lining does not get the message to stabilize and strengthen and so may begin to shed before the end of the "usual" 28 day cycle. Women's periods can get shorter and shorter as a result. A sure sign of no follicle being released (anovulation) is when a woman who has had regular periods most of her cycling life begin to see cycle shorten to 25, 24, 23, days in length.

However, periods may not necessarily get shorter. Both progesterone and estradiol send messages to the same cells – but the messages are significantly different. Estradiol sends the message to the cells of the uterus to grow the lining ready for implantation. Progesterone sends the message to stop growing and start developing and maturing to prepare for a possible pregnancy. If there is no progesterone surge to cancel the message to grow the lining of the uterus, then estradiol can become the dominant hormone messenger. Its message is to "grow cells" and as a result, the uterine lining can continue to grow, getting thicker and richer in cells and blood. This can result in a sensation of swelling and bloating. When shedding finally starts, periods then can become painful and heavy. One of progesterone's effects is to decrease uterine muscle contractions by promoting uterine muscle relaxation, a lack of progesterone can therefore result in an increase in the intensity of menstrual cramps.

Estradiol also sends messages to the breast tissue to grow. Breast cells increase in number and rate of multiplication under the influence of estradiol. Once again, progesterone is that natural counterbalance and sends messages to the breast cells to decrease breast cell growth and reduce the rate of multiplication. Progesterone also promotes normal cell death in the breast tissue which is important in the prevention of cancer. In perimenopause if estradiol is sending the message to breast cells to grow and that message is unchecked by the non-occurrence of the expected surge in progesterone, then breast cell growth will continue. This can cause discomfort, leading to tender, sore and swollen breasts in the second half of the monthly cycle. Because the breast cells store fat, any growth in the number of breast cells will increase the amount of fat stored in the breasts and breast size can grow significantly during perimenopause. Another possible unwelcome side effect during perimenopause is bloating. Aldosterone is another hormone in the body and it promotes water retention and swelling. Progesterone blocks the receptors for aldosterone and thus allows normal fluid loss and decreases swelling.

Thyroid hormone is important for regulating the body's metabolism, the utilization of fat stores, and calcium balance. Estrogen may decrease the function of thyroid hormone as it can increase the production of Thyroid Binding Globulin which binds to the thyroid hormone making it inactive and unavailable to be used in the body, thereby decreasing metabolism and increasing fat deposits. Progesterone is the natural counterbalance to estrogen, it decreases thyroid binding globulin and therefore increases the activity of circulating thyroid hormone.

Estrogen Dominance

As is probably becoming clear, there is a fine balance between levels of estradiol and progesterone, and practitioners want to make sure there is a good balance between the two hormones. Too much estradiol in relation to progesterone is likely to result in some of the symptoms of Estrogen Dominance or "Progesterone Deficiency" listed in the next diagram.

Symptoms of Estrogen Dominance	
Accelerated aging	Weight gain
Anxiety	Breast Tenderness
Bloating	Decreased libido
Increased risk of blood clots	Fibrocystic breasts
Increased risk of breast cancer	Uterine Fibroids
Increased risk of gallstones	Food cravings
Increased risk of post-partum depression	Headaches
Irregular menses	Heavy Menstrual Periods
Irritability	Hypersensitivity
Mood Swings	Increased triglycerides
Ovarian cysts	

Although women of any age can become estrogen dominant, it can be especially evident during perimenopause and menopause, when reproductive hormones are supposed to take a natural downturn. There is a misconception that the symptoms of menopause are normal. They may be common, but they're not normal. Today, many women are experiencing eight to ten years (or more), of life-disrupting perimenopausal mayhem. It was not meant to be this way, we were meant to see some mild symptoms leading up to menopause. It is only in the last twenty years or so that symptoms of perimenopause have become so significant.

Estrogen also affects the brain. If estrogen is too high (or low), depression, anxiety, insomnia, decreased sex drive and reduced concentration can occur. GABA is an amino acid that is a inhibitory neurotransmitter. Progesterone also activates the GABA receptor sites making GABA more effective. Progesterone is a natural antidepressant and can help prevent anxiety.

Fiber is a great aid to reducing estrogen dominance because waste estrogens bind to fiber and leave the body via the normal route. If fiber in the diet is low, then there is little for the waste estrogens to bind to and they end up passing back into the blood stream and recirculate estrogen in the body. Ensuring adequate fiber and maintaining regular and frequent bowel movements helps remove waste estrogens from the body.

When you have your hormones tested in saliva, the lab results should calculate the ratio between progesterone and estradiol. The ideal balance is 20:1. If necessary, your practitioner will be able to help you use bioidentical hormones to make sure your estradiol and progesterone levels are balanced correctly so that your symptoms are lessened and, hopefully, go away completely.

Infertility and Polycystic Ovarian Syndrome (PCOS)

PCOS is a condition linked to the way the body processes insulin after it has been produced by the pancreas to regulate blood sugar (glucose). As mentioned earlier, insulin is the key that opens the door on the cell wall to allow glucose inside to be used for energy. We are still genetically "wired" to eat nutrient-rich foods and a diet low in simpole carbohydrates and sustain much greater levels of movement and exercise. With many modern diets that are high in simple carbohydrates combined with not as much exercise, blood sugar is often high and so insulin is often elevated to try to manage blood sugar levels. Too much insulin over time damages the ability of the body's cells to properly utilize insulin to convert glucose to energy. This process creates Insulin Resistance. Some people may have a genetic predisposition to Insulin Resistance, while others develop the condition through high stress and unhealthy lifestyle choices.

Insulin Resistance significantly reduces the insulin sensitivity of cells, which slows the processing of glucose through the cell wall for conversion to energy. Insulin will no longer act as the key to the door to allow glucose into the cell. As a result, glucose remains in the blood stream, causing elevated levels of blood sugar. Because this is dangerous for the body, the excess glucose is sent to the liver. Once there, the glucose is converted into glycogen, and sent off in the blood stream to be stored throughout the body. This process can lead to weight gain.

Too much insulin circulating also stimulates the ovaries and the adrenal gland to produce larger amounts of testosterone, which may prevent the ovaries from releasing a follicle each month, thus contributing to infertility. The follicles may begin to develop one per month, but the presence of higher levels of testosterone than normal will signal to the body that ovulation should not occur. So it doesn't. This means that there are a growing number of half-grown follicles in the ovary which become cysts – hence the name Poly (many) Cystic (cysts). High levels of insulin can also increase the conversion of DHEA to estradiol which creates a situation where the body has too much estradiol that is not balanced out by progesterone. The balance between all the hormones is gradually upset which has a further effect on weight gain, the formation of further cystic follicles or ovarian cysts, and mood imbalance.

There are several symptoms of PCOS, including irregular or completely absent periods, obesity, acne, depression, exhaustion, lack of mental alertness, excessive facial or body hair, male pattern hair loss, obesity, acne, skin tags, decreased sex drive. Because the symptoms vary so widely and not all women display all the symptoms, conventional practitioners can misdiagnose PCOS which is a problem because studies show that women suffering from PCOS have a higher risk of coronary heart disease and Type 2 Diabetes.

A practitioner skilled in understanding the intricacies of metabolism and its impact on hormone balance can recognize symptoms of PCOS and confirm its diagnosis in a couple of different ways. Testing hormones in saliva is a quick and effective way to identify if PCOS may exist. Elevated testosterone levels will show in salivary hormone test years before a serum test for testosterone will register an increase in testosterone. This is because saliva testing measures the bioavailable levels of hormones circulating in the body, whereas serum testing measures the total levels of hormone circulating. Saliva hormone testing will also measure levels of Progesterone, and Estradiol.

Some practitioners will order an ultrasound of the uterus and ovaries to see if the ovaries are polycystic, although polycystic ovaries aren't technically required for a PCOS diagnosis. Polycystic ovaries can be up to twice the size of normal ovaries and so show up well on an ultrasound. Other testing can include checking fasting glucose and insulin levels, a glucose tolerance test, and other tests to rule out disorders similar to PCOS.

Treatment for PCOS can include a combination of the following: nutritional supplementation, lifestyle changes, a realistic exercise program, bioidentical hormone supplementation, diet that is rich in lean protein and low on carbohydrates, and perhaps medication that can help lower insulin levels if needed. If you have PCOS, a practitioner will be able to help you take some important steps in correcting the problem, adding things to lifestyle and diet that will help, as well as supporting the gradual shift away from foods and activities that contribute to PCOS.

Testosterone and DHEA Deficiency

The adrenal glands continue to produce some testosterone and DHEA throughout the lifespan, but the amount produced is greatly reduced the older we get. How well the adrenal gland is working is linked closely to how well the ovaries are working. This is because in the developing embryo, the group of cells that develop into the ovaries (or testes in male babies) is also the starting point for part of the adrenal gland. As the embryo develops, the two groups of cells migrate to the two difference places. Hormone signals sent to the ovaries also send hormone signals to the adrenal gland because both glands come from the same "starting material". It is however, well established that the ovaries continue to produce testosterone at a relatively stable rate in menopausal years, and may even increase production.

Testosterone drops as we age, by age forty there is usually about half the amount of testosterone we had in our twenties. Most testosterone comes from DHEA, and DHEA starts to drop in our thirties. That means that if DHEA drops, so does testosterone. Enzymes are necessary to convert cholesterol to DHEA and then convert DHEA to testosterone. As enzyme levels drop with age, the rate of conversion declines and so contributes to lower testosterone levels. The number of testosterone receptors (docking stations) can also decline with time, and this can reduce how much circulating testosterone can be used. We are all individuals so there is no one set path that any person will follow in changes to hormone levels. Some people have the genetic predisposition to keep them vital for many more years than others. This is why testing is so important. Because our individual genetic codes are all so different, your practitioner needs to know what is happening with YOU.

Hysterectomy and Oophorectomy (removal of the ovaries)

The topic of hysterectomy is a big one – and beyond the scope of this book, but it is important to note that approximately six hundred thousand hysterectomies are performed annually in the United States making it the second most frequently performed major surgical procedure in the United States. An estimated twenty million American women have had a hysterectomy and nearly half of the women who have their ovaries removed, no matter what their age, are likely to develop immediate testosterone deficiency due to the total loss of ovarian testosterone.

There is an increasing awareness that many hysterectomies are avoidable, so when considering a hysterectomy, find a practitioner to work with who is skilled in the use of bioidentical hormone balancing – there are plenty of options to look at before having a hysterectomy or an oophorectomy. If the uterus is removed and the ovaries are left in place – there is still an increased likelihood of changing patterns of hormone production. The artery that leads to the uterus may be the source for up to two-thirds of the ovaries' blood supply, so when surgical removal of the uterus disrupts the blood supply, the ovaries may stop functioning. In addition, the uterus produces chemicals, known as prostaglandins that send cyclic hormone messages to the ovaries. If the uterus is removed, this rhythm is disrupted and this, in turn, can result in the earlier development of testosterone deficiency.

Metabolic Syndrome – Too much Testosterone and DHEA

Is it possible to have too much testosterone and DHEA – the androgen hormones? Yes. As we saw in the discussion of PCOS, high insulin levels and insulin resistance can cause testosterone to increase, resulting in a host of symptoms including male pattern baldness, facial hair growth, acne, skin tags and more. In younger women, the impact can reduce fertility. Infertility is less of an issue for women in their forties and beyond, however, the implications for long term health are just as relevant for older women as they are for younger women. When testosterone is elevated in any woman as measured by salivary hormone testing – it is an indicator of possible insulin resistance; it suggests that the body is producing high levels of insulin which are not being effectively used by the body. Insulin resistance is the starting point for Metabolic Syndrome and later Type Two Diabetes. The word "Diabetes" doesn't sound as scary as "Cancer", and yet it is a disease that is just as powerful a killer. Diabetes may not kill as fast as cancer can, but there are so many complications and impacts on a life lived with diabetes, that we should all be determined to do what we can to beat diabetes – just as we are determined to beat cancer.

Can testosterone be high and there still be low libido?

Yes! Without a doubt. A woman who has high testosterone as a result of insulin resistance is also likely to have greater weight gain, increased stress, chronic fatigue, estrogen dominance, progesterone deficiency, tender breasts, and hot flashes. Who could feel sexy with that going on?

Low Estrogen

Hot flashes are one of the most common symptoms discussed in connection with menopause. Even teenagers have heard of hot flashes. For some women approaching the natural ending of reproductive lifespan, estrogen levels do begin to fall. This means there is no hormone signal to thicken the lining of the uterus, and as the follicles are depleted, there is no ovulation. With no thickening of the uterine lining, menstrual flow reduces, becomes irregular and eventually stops. The brain however is still signaling the need to produce estradiol and progesterone. When no (or not enough) hormone is produced, the natural feedback loop has the brain signaling "make estradiol, make progesterone, make estradiol, ovulate, dammit, ovulate".

This heightened communication activity in the brain, in the hypothalamus to be exact, stimulates activity in the vasomotor center next door. The vasomotor center controls capillary dilation and sweating and so, when stimulated by the panicking hypothalamus, it is thrown off balance and becomes hyperactive, signaling the need to cool the body down. The body cools itself by dilating the capillaries to allow more blood to flow to the skin surface and be cooled by air. Under pressure to deliver rapid air conditioning, this dilation of the capillaries with blood rushing to the surface makes the skin red and flushed, and it also causes the surge of heat felt all over the skin as a result of the mad panic to send the heat outwards to the exterior of the body. Hence a Hot Flash with reddened blushing skin! Next, having sent a lot of the body's heat outwards, the body core temperature can drop quickly, and a woman is then left feeling cold and shivery. You can spot a postmenopausal woman who is not on hormone supplementation, she dresses in layers and never goes anywhere without a fan and an extra jacket.

There are plenty of women who don't get hot flashes, who don't experience the feedback loop to the hypothalamus screaming for more estrogen and progesterone. These women usually have diets rich in fresh vegetables and vitamin C that encourage natural production of progesterone. Even though there is less estrogen being produced with menopause, as long as progesterone is present, the hypothalamus gets the messages that enough hormones are present to keep it calm and collected. Supplementing with the right amounts of topical bioidentical progesterone can be an excellent method for controlling hot flashes. Make sure your practitioner tests your hormones in saliva though – you want to make sure you have the right amount of any supplementation, more is not necessarily better, balance is what you want to achieve.

Incontinence

Really?? Sorry ladies – yes, low estrogen can also contribute to another significant health issue. Estrogen is important for maintaining the health of vaginal tissue. Loss of strength and tone in the vaginal muscles increases significantly with menopause. This can result in both incontinence (urine leakage) and vaginal dryness. Women are twice more likely to suffer from urinary incontinence than men, and an estimated one in three women over the age of sixty are likely to have bladder control problems.

For many women, these issues start to occur with perimenopause, although changes in weight and pelvic surgeries can also contribute to incontinence problems. The pelvic floor is a collection of many small muscles woven together like a basket that supports the bladder and uterus. As women age, gain weight, have children, or undergo hysterectomy, it is common for this "basket" to drop as a result of decreased muscle strength. When this happens, incontinence and decreased vaginal sensation may become lingering health concerns. Kegel exercises for the pelvic floor can be done with or without vaginal weights and, when performed consistently, can help prevent and/or treat decreased vaginal tone and the issues that may accompany it, including incontinence – specifically stress incontinence. Stress incontinence occurs along with physical stress such as running, sneezing, laughing or coughing.

Stress incontinence tends to increase with age and is a particularly common complaint in postmenopausal years. While toning exercises can be very effective, estrogen is essential for maintaining the tone of the vaginal tissues and muscles. A comprehensive treatment plan for stress incontinence should include strengthening exercises along with proper hormone balancing to ensure adequate muscle tone. Many women may benefit from estrogen supplementation, and specifically from estriol cream applied directly onto vaginal tissue, especially if used within the first year that symptoms are experienced. If this is something you are beginning to notice, it can be embarrassing to mention this symptom to your practitioner, but if you don't, how can your practitioner help you?

Cortisol

Cortisol is secreted in the adrenal glands and provides the chemical message to influence the following functions.

- Initiate the waking response in the morning
- Increase the breakdown of stored fatty tissue into glycerol and fatty acids (to create energy) when needed
- Ensure proper glucose metabolism
- Regulate blood pressure
- Initiation of insulin release for blood sugar balancing
- Immune function
- Anti-Inflammatory response
- Control the fight or flight response.

In a healthy person cortisol has a regular daily pattern shown in the next diagram. During sleep, cortisol levels are low. Just before awakening, cortisol levels begin to rise. Cortisol is necessary to kick start the body for the day. As the melatonin controlled night time "fast" comes to an end, cortisol is produced to bring the body and brain to a state of alertness in preparation for the day. Surfacing from sleep, cortisol begins to surge from the adrenal gland and is distributed via the blood stream to the various parts of the body that have receptors ready and waiting. Energy is needed to get out of bed and begin movement and thinking, so cortisol is produced to convert stored fat into usable energy.

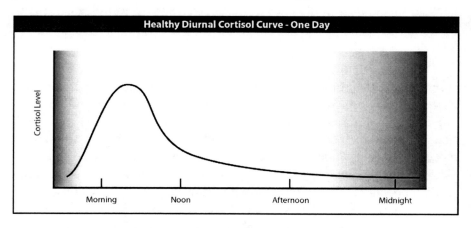

Blood pressure drops during sleep, so cortisol heads off to be delivered to the receptors that influence blood pressure. Cortisol rises ready for management of the fight or flight response as well as all the metabolic functions. Back in the cave dwelling days the transition from sleep to waking was potentially dangerous in terms of predators being alerted by waking movements, so cortisol is released to increase awareness. All these and more functions kick into gear when wakening from sleep and that is why there should be a steep rise in cortisol levels within the first thirty minutes after awakening. This is called the Cortisol Awakening Response and cortisol level should be at its highest for the whole day at this point.

The first order of the day is to find food. Now that melatonin has dropped, appetite will rise. As breakfast is digested (releasing glucose into the blood stream), insulin will be released from the pancreas to begin managing the glucose. As the day progresses, cortisol levels begin to drop as the need for the "jump start" passes and other body functions take over. By bedtime cortisol levels are low again, approaching the low levels of the night before. As cortisol drops, the awake functions begin to close down, the body and brain get tired and it is time to go to bed. Turning out the light and settling to sleep will signal melatonin to rise and cortisol levels to continue to drop, thus lowering blood pressure and demand for energy (glucose).

The adrenal gland also controls the fight or flight response. In cave dwelling times this fight or flight response was stimulated by activities such as a predatory reptile or mammal getting a little too close; or mothers observing their toddlers about to pick poisonous berries; warring tribes approaching with spears; getting stuck in the pathway of a rampaging wooly mammoth. In modern times we have different stressors: the minutes when a child wanders off out of sight in a store; when we drive past a police car at fifteen miles over the speed limit racing to get to work; sounds of footsteps behind us on a dark night; the oven bursting into flames, along with dinner. Whatever the stressor or threat, the cortisol response is the same:

1. The autonomic nervous system automatically puts the body on alert.

2. The adrenal gland automatically releases the stress hormones, cortisol and epinephrine (adrenaline).

3. The heart automatically beats harder and more rapidly.

4. Breathing automatically becomes more rapid.

5. The thyroid gland automatically stimulates the metabolism.

6. Larger muscles automatically receive more oxygenated blood.

The elevated cortisol levels that come with the stress response will also provide heightened memory functions, a burst of increased immunity (in case of wounding), and lower sensitivity to pain. The brain can make the decision to fight, freeze, or run away; whichever way – the body automatically primes ready for the action that is chosen. After the stressor passes, the body returns to normal: stress hormone secretion drops, heart rate and breathing slow, metabolism adjusts and muscles relax.

While cortisol is an important and helpful part of the body's response to stress, it is also important that the body's relaxation response is activated so the body's functions can, in fact, return to normal following a stressful event. Unfortunately, in the current high-stress culture, the body's stress response is activated so often that the body doesn't always have a chance to return to normal, resulting in a state of chronic stress; there is much more on this in the chapter on Stress.

A frequently asked question about cortisol is "Does cortisol make you fat?" The answer is no, eating too much of the wrong thing and not exercising makes you fat. However, imbalances in cortisol do have significant impacts on metabolism. Too much cortisol can decrease thyroid function – and the thyroid gland is vital for controlling metabolism. Too little cortisol can influence blood sugar (glucose) metabolism. Both of these imbalances can contribute to significant weight gain.

Hormones and Depression

Hormone fluctuations can have an impact on mood, and mood disorders vary significantly in duration and severity. Hormones work in partnership with neurotransmitters, the chemical messengers found primarily in the brain. Hormones, particularly estradiol and progesterone, have a direct impact on the creation, release, activity and breakdown of neurotransmitters. Neurotransmitters that impact mood are Serotonin, GABA, Dopamine, Norepinephrine, Epinephrine and Glutamate. Serotonin and GABA are what are known as inhibitory neurotransmitters, they inhibit (restrain) some brain activity and have a calming effect. Serotonin is also associated with the feeling of being connected to community, of being valued and loved. GABA is nature's valium and it helps to have enough to settle to sleep at night. Progesterone is an agonist to GABA, so having adequate levels of progesterone can help ensure the brain can make enough GABA. Postmenopausal women whose progesterone levels have declined can sometimes find it hard to relax and sleep because of reduced sensitivity to GABA.

Dopamine is one of the feel good neurotransmitters. Human brains evolved to give us pleasure when we do something that promotes survival and increases the ability to pass on our genetic code – including eating and having sex. When we do something that achieves those goals we get a little squirt of happiness in the form of dopamine. Testosterone and DHEA support the production of dopamine, and estrogen helps modulate dopamine so it stays balanced. So, if sex hormone levels are declining, then it may be that dopamine levels are also declining. The little boosts of dopamine induced happiness get fewer and farther apart and mood can suffer as a result.

Someone having trouble sleeping, trouble getting to sleep or staying asleep, trouble with racing thoughts that go on and on in endless circles, may benefit from testing neurotransmitter levels in addition to hormone levels. A poor night's sleep could be the result of a number of imbalances: low cortisol, high cortisol, low GABA, low progesterone, high glutamate, high norepinephrine or epinephrine. Testing gives the practitioner key biochemical indicators to match with symptoms and good information from which to recommend the approach that will solve the sleep problem sooner rather than later.

Testing – Evaluating Hormone Levels

A good starting place for assessing hormonal status is to measure estradiol, progesterone, testosterone, DHEA, and also cortisol levels at four times during the day. Remember: cortisol has a well-established twenty-four hour diurnal rhythm, and the times of day when it is measured will reveal unique aspects of health. This individualized approach of bioidentical hormone treatment requires a saliva hormone test. Unlike serum tests which reflect total levels, including the large bound portion, saliva testing will measure only active (free/unbound) hormone levels. Measuring inactive hormone levels has very limited utility in assessing function or balance. When testing the sex hormones through saliva, it is also important to assess adrenal status (DHEA and diurnal cortisols). Even if the chief complaints seem to be an imbalance of the sex hormones, hormone pathways are so closely linked that an imbalance in one area will affect the function and efficiency of another.

{ HRT or BHRT }

The difference between bioidentical and synthetic hormones starts at the molecular level. Bioidentical hormones have the exact same chemical structure as hormones made by the human body, and can replicate the actions of those made naturally. Side effects and risk factors are minimized when your body recognizes its own molecular structure, fills its receptor sites efficiently, and can utilize, break down, and detoxify hormones effectively.

Synthetic hormones, on the other hand, have an altered molecular structure that the body does not recognize completely, thus their actions are not straightforward and they are not detoxified from the body as easily. Side effects are common with these types of hormones because they are foreign to the body.

Bioidentical hormones can be customized to meet the individual needs of each person using them for supplementation. Synthetic hormones, however, are prescribed as a "one size fits all", and cannot be specifically made for an individual.

Sex hormones identical to human (bioidentical) hormones have been available for over 50 years. Pharmaceutical companies, however, prefer synthetic hormones. Synthetic hormones (not found in nature) can be patented, whereas real (natural, bioidentical) hormones can not. Patented drugs are more profitable than non-patented drugs. Sex hormone prescription sales have made billions of dollars for pharmaceutical companies.

When the Women's Health Initiative, a long term health study of postmenopausal women indicated that incidences of breast cancer, heart disease and osteoporosis increase with the use of some Synthetic hormones, the study was halted. Women wanted a safe alternative to hormone supplementation and the use of natural bioidentical hormone supplementation has been on the rise ever since.

Even though many forms of bioidentical hormone supplementation are manufactured in a lab – it is important to understand that the chemical structure of these products matches exactly the chemical structure of the hormones made naturally in the body.

It is critical however, when using any hormone supplementation, that you test your hormones to measure the bioidentical levels that currently exist in your body. Your practitioner will need this information to make sure that your treatment plan fits your needs exactly. Testing bioavailable levels of hormones in saliva is the key to successful bioidentical hormone supplementation.

Methods of hormone supplementation

While any form of BHRT is a step in the right direction when your hormones are imbalanced, certain methods may work better for you than others. There are various delivery methods for bioidentical hormones which may include hormone creams, gels, patches, sublingual tablets, injections and pellet insertion. Each person is different and their needs may change over time. This is why it is important to have an individualized program designed for each woman experiencing symptoms of perimenopause or menopause.

Method	Advantages	Disadvantages
Transdermal creams	Goes straight to tissue without passing through liver, doses can be lower. Customizable to each person	Sticky, possible to contaminate surfaces in the home and affect family
Pellets	Can be implanted for 3-4 month periods, convenient	Soreness at implant site
Sublingual	Simplicity. Goes straight to tissue without passing through liver.	Can be swallowed reducing effectiveness of dose. Can have a bitter taste.
Oral	Simplicity	Passes through the liver first so doses have to be higher
Patch	Convenience of applying once a week. Offers a more steady flow of hormones.	If patches fall off , they are hard to stick back on. There may be an allergic reaction to the glue

Chapter Two Summary – Hormones

- The endocrine system, how hormones work
- Progesterone, Estrogens, DHEA, Testosterone, Cortisol
- Changes in the cycle with perimenopause
- Polycystic Ovarian Syndrome
- Metabolic Syndrome
- The role of cortisol
- Hormones and mood
- Testing hormone levels
- Hormone supplementation options

CHAPTER THREE

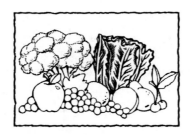

NUTRITION

I have been fortunate to travel to a range of different cities in the US in the course of my work. I like new places and I absolutely love to fly. As a former geography teacher, if the sky is clear I can easily spend the entire journey across the whole country looking out of the window just absorbing the geography below me. When it comes to eating on these trips however, I frequently find myself needing to forage like a Neanderthal for food that will work for my body. Managing dairy, gluten, and (I reluctantly accept) egg intolerances, means most airline food is off limits; airport food is fast and oil soaked; cheese permeates all salads; and a plateful of breaded meat or fish would leave me doubled over in pain. As I eat pretty healthily, I eventually found that in certain parts of the country it is just easier to go to the grocery store than try local delicacies that will be loaded with butter, bread and cheese. Over time, I evolved my travel back-ups that have saved me from hunger on many an occasion – avocados, salmon, apples, nuts, protein bars, and plenty of green tea bags. Ah yes, the high life of business travel!

There is now a wealth of information about nutrition available everywhere. From diet books to web articles, everyone seems to have an opinion about what you should be eating. It is no secret that good nutrition plays an essential role in maintaining health. While you already know it is important to eat a healthy diet, you may find it more difficult to sort through all of the information about nutrition and food choices and decide what is right for you. In addition, for some people, eating food is simply a necessary activity to provide the body with fuel, for others it can be the high points of the day onto which great attention and effort is focused. Everyone is somewhere on the spectrum between these two points of view.

The right food for your body is one of the best medicines there is. Nourishing your body with the vitamins, minerals, and substances it needs to be healthy is the single most positive thing you can do to care for yourself. Conversely, the wrong foods can have significant impact on your overall level of health, bringing on discomfort, pain, chronic disease and weight gain, all of which can have a knock-on effect on many systems in your body – the heart, liver, kidney, spleen, gallbladder, joints and so on.

What drives us to eat? Because the body needs food for fuel and survival, there has to be a mechanism that ensures that we eat. There are in fact, dozens of chemical messengers in the mouth, the stomach, the intestines, liver and bloodstream, all geared to make sure we eat. Some of these messengers work in the short term around one particular meal; and others, as we know, work in the long term, ensuring we maintain enough fat supplies for seasonal variations. The hypothalamus is a key area of the brain that controls hunger, appetite and satiety (the feeling of being full). It also adjusts metabolism, the rate at which the body uses or stores food and energy stores.

Two major hormones control the desire to eat. As mentioned in the Chapter on Sleep, leptin is a hormone that modulates appetite and metabolic rate and is made in the fat cells. Leptin is released into the body in proportion to the amount of fat cells you have and seems to be the feedback mechanism that tells the body that fat stores are adequate, so there is no need to eat. When fat stores decline, leptin will signal the body to eat more at each meal to rebuild the stores. This very sophisticated and ancient survival mechanism can make keeping weight off difficult in modern times.

The major hormone that influences actual feelings of hunger is ghrelin. Ghrelin is made in the lining of the stomach and upper small intestine and stimulates the brain to send "I'm hungry" messages. It is an appetite stimulant, and levels usually peak right before we eat. Lowest levels are found about an hour after eating. It is important to know that it is not your empty stomach that stimulates ghrelin production – it is actually your brain anticipating a meal. If you are used to eating four meals a day – ghrelin levels will rise four times each day as you think about the approaching meal time. If you eat twice a day – there will be two surges of ghrelin. The amount of ghrelin per surge increases if you only eat twice a day – making sure you are really hungry both those two times.

What is it that bodies are looking for when the hormone ghrelin is released? We know there are three main types of nutrients – proteins, carbohydrates and fats. We hear about them all the time, but we will take another look here in the context of making choices to use food as best medicine.

Protein

Protein is an essential component of diet; to go without protein invites trouble and possible death. Proteins are the largest and most complex molecules in the body and are made up of chains of amino acids. There are at least twenty two different amino acids which form together in a limitless number of chain configurations. To give you an idea of the scale, each protein molecule can contain about nine hundred amino acids. Proteins are enzymes (catalysts that make actions happen faster) and, because every single molecular event in every single cell in the body is regulated by enzymes, proteins are essential for the body to function. We go through our day, often barely conscious of all the billions of cells in our body. We don't really need to think about those billions of cells all busily doing whatever it is they need to do – respiring, converting and using energy, transmitting chemical messages, and so on, all that happens without us paying attention to it, and it happens because we have proteins in the body to make it happen.

Proteins are also important for making sure that blood will clot, that oxygen and carbon dioxide is transported around the body, for the build-up and maintenance of muscles, skin, veins, arteries and tendons. Antibodies that defend against disease are proteins, as are the particles that carry fat and cholesterol around the body. Proteins are vital to cellular function, to life itself. Without the daily protein requirement, the body begins to deteriorate. Unlike fats and carbohydrates which are stored as fat, proteins do not last forever. Each protein has a definite lifespan – some minutes, some months. Think about what happens when someone breaks a leg. That leg has to be immobilized for weeks, often months, while the bone heals. During the period of immobilization, the muscle in the leg gradually wastes away as the protein stored in the muscle is steadily broken down by natural recycling processes. After the cast is removed, it takes hard work to rebuild the muscle to its former strong state. We lose protein every day, all the time, as the body is performing billions of necessary cell functions. It is vital that the body is supplied with adequate protein to maintain healthy body functioning.

How is protein made?

Our individual genetic code provides the blue print for making proteins. The genetic code determines how those twenty two amino acids are strung together, in what order, in what chain length and for what function.

The amino acids are building blocks of protein molecules and they come from two sources. The first source is food. Protein in food is broken down by specialized digestive enzymes in the digestive tract. There are a group of digestive enzymes in the stomach, and then another group in the small (upper) intestine. These enzymes begin to break down the large proteins into smaller and smaller proteins, until eventually only the amino acids are left. The amino acids are then absorbed through the gut wall and taken to the liver. The liver is the key organ where new protein is made. The newly formed proteins then head out in the bloodstream to various parts of the body to be used, for example, in the muscles of the heart.

The second source of proteins is from the body itself. The body can make some amino acids from the byproducts of carbohydrate metabolism. However, only some of the twenty two amino acids can be made by the body, and these are called collectively the non-essential amino acids. The remaining amino acids are known as essential amino acids because it is essential that we get them from diet. Some food proteins have the correct balance of amino acids, for example, meat, milk, eggs; others are not as complete, for example, soy is missing methionine, cereals do not have lysine.

The diagram below shows the names of the essential and nonessential amino acids:

Essential Amino Acids		Non-Essential Amino Acids	
Histadine	Threonine	Alanine	Glycine*
Isoleucine	Tryptophan	Arganine*	Proline*
Leucine	Valine Serine*	Aspartic Acid	Serine*
Lysine Cysteine*	Tyrosine*	Cysteine*	Tyrosine*
Methionine	Asparagine*	Glutamic Acid	Asparagine*
Phenylalanine	Seleocysteine	Glutamine*	Selenocysteine

Obtained From Nutrition   *Under Certain Conditions   Synthesized By The Body

Carbohydrate

Carbohydrate's major function is providing enough energy to a variety of tissues, especially to the brain and the nervous system, both of which cannot utilize other nutrients for energy. Carbohydrates do not contribute to the structure of tissues or control molecular events like proteins do. Carbohydrates do contribute to the regulation of metabolism.

Carbohydrate is usually starch from bread, potatoes, rice, pasta, but also comes from all vegetables and fruits, sucrose from sugar, and lactose from milk. Starches are made up of large glucose molecules stuck together. These large glucose molecules are very easily digested into smaller individual glucose units which are then very easily absorbed into the blood stream. Lactose and sucrose are much smaller units digested by the enzymes lactase and sucrase and then sent to the liver. Just about everyone can digest sucrose, but a significant number of people cannot digest lactose and are therefore lactose intolerant. Undigested lactose is passed from the small intestine into the large intestine where bacteria ferment the lactose which then causes gas, digestive upsets and diarrhea. If you experience the above symptoms on a regular basis, it could be a good idea to mention that to your practitioner. Lactose is found in dairy products and anyone who is lactose intolerant has an allergy to milk/dairy products. There is more to read about food allergies later in this chapter.

Under normal conditions, most carbohydrates in a meal are broken down to glucose and as a result, glucose levels in the blood measured before and after eating show big differences. A meal high in carbohydrates, such as a breakfast of pancakes with syrup, will create a high level of blood glucose, because the large glucose molecules are broken down very quickly. The peak in blood glucose occurs about half an hour after eating and then levels of glucose drop again by about an hour after eating. The body maintains blood glucose levels within narrow ranges using the hormones insulin and glucagon which are made in the pancreas. Insulin is secreted when blood glucose levels rise and its main job is to remove excess glucose from the bloodstream. In the liver, insulin then converts the glucose molecule from a carbohydrate to a fat. The actual molecular structure of glucose is changed and this makes it possible for the new fat molecule to be stored in the body ready for later use. In muscle, the glucose is chemically altered to a different kind of carbohydrate – glycogen, which acts as a special short term energy supply for muscular activity such as walking and running. As a young teenager, I hiked regularly in the mountains with my father. On the steep uphill sections, he would strategically slip a small candy bar in my hand; he knew that munching on that bar would give me the energy to make it to the top as I chewed and the glucose was released. I wasn't thinking about the science, I just loved the sweet and salty chocolate and nut combination that took my mind off how steep the trail was!

If for some reason there is no further supply of carbohydrate, the body has another mechanism to make sure there is enough blood glucose. When blood glucose levels begin to drop to the lower range, then the hormone glucagon is released. Glucagon signals the body to switch from burning carbs for energy to burning fat for energy, releasing glycogen to glucose. Long distance runners will eat lots of carbohydrate the day before a race to provide lots of glucose for the first part of the run. Once the circulating glucose is used up, then the body releases glucagon to start burning fat cells to release stored energy. When my father ran out of candy bars and there were still a couple of hours left to hike, my body had to switch to burning fat to get me through the last few miles. Now when I hike, I will have a good breakfast to get me going, and after that, work on burning my fat supplies.

Fats

Fats are interesting. There is so much information in the media about fat in diet: essential fatty acids, high fat, low fat, milk fat, omega 3s, omega 6's, saturated fat, mono-unsaturated fat, fish oils and on and on. It can be a challenge to make sense of the story on fat and work out what are the right fats to eat.

Some important chemical facts about fat. First – fats are not soluble in water, we know that because oil left over in a frying pan needs detergent to break up the fat molecules to clean it. Secondly – some fats are solid at room temperature e.g. butter; and others are liquid at room temperature e.g. olive oil. We need to keep these two facts in mind when we look at the structure and usage of fat in the body.

The basic structure of fat is fatty acids and they come grouped together in threes. Fat molecules are called triglycerides (tri= three) and are composed of a glycerol molecule with three fatty acids attached (think of three kids on a skateboard). Like proteins which can use the amino acids to make any sort of chain, triglycerides can use any combination of different types of fatty acids to make a fat molecule.

There are three types of fat molecule: saturated, mono-unsaturated and poly-unsaturated fatty acids. Most fats are made up of a combination of saturated and unsaturated fat – with one being the more dominant. Olive oil for example is largely mono-unsaturated fat, but has poly-unsaturated and saturated fats as well.

- Saturated fats are solid at room temperature and are found mainly in animal and dairy products, but are also found in coconuts and palm kernels. A small amount of saturated fat can be beneficial to the health of the immune system and digestive tract.

- Mono-unsaturated fats are liquid at room temperature and solid when refrigerated. Olive, canola and peanut oils are high in mono-unsaturated fats, as are avocados, almonds, pecans, peanuts, and cashews.

- Poly-unsaturated fats are liquid at room temperature and when refrigerated. They are unstable (the chemical bonds between the molecules are weak), can go rancid quickly and should not be used for cooking. Examples include fish oils and most vegetable and seed oils. There are two types of poly-unsaturated fats that are essential because the body cannot make them – Omega 3 and Omega 6. Omega 3 fats are found in ocean fish, grass fed meats, free range poultry and eggs. Omega 3 fatty acids are helpful in protecting against blood clots, heart disease, high blood pressure, diabetes, colitis and inflammatory diseases. Omega 6 fatty acids are found in vegetable, sunflower, peanut and other nut and seed oils. Both fatty acids are helpful, however current guidelines suggest that you should have significantly more Omega 3 than Omega 6 oils in your diet.

{ Trans Fatty Acids }

Trans fatty acids were invented to give foods a longer shelf life. Polyunsaturated fats are superheated and then have extra hydrogen atoms added. This change to the chemical structure of the fatty acid means the fat is solid at room temperature and therefore less likely to go rancid and spoil. Although people often like the texture of goods baked and cooked with trans fats, the body has a hard time processing them. Because the chemical structure of the fats has been altered, the body does not recognize these fats correctly. Human cell membranes are made up of a combination of fatty acids and proteins – but mainly fatty acids. Cell membranes composed of trans fats cannot function optimally. The normal biochemical processes do not happen at the correct rate in the correct way because the trans fat blocks the mechanism. No trans fats are essential fatty acids; in fact, the consumption of trans fats increases the risk of coronary heart disease by raising levels of "bad" LDL cholesterol and lowering levels of "good" HDL cholesterol. Health authorities worldwide recommend that consumption of trans fat be reduced to trace amounts. Trans fats from partially hydrogenated oils are more harmful than naturally occurring oils.

Trans fats are often found in: Chips, Processed foods, Baked goods, Pudding.

Fats are digested by the enzyme lipase, and lipase is found in the watery fluids in the gut. However, we know that oil and water don't mix, so a third agent is needed to disperse the fat into small molecules. That agent is bile. Bile is made in the liver and distributed through the gall bladder. Bile is a powerful "detergent" and its presence permits the fat molecules that we eat to be broken down by the enzyme lipase. The broken down fat molecules then pass through the gut wall into the blood stream and are transported to their destination. It is really important to have a healthy liver and a working gall bladder – without that, your body struggles to digest fat.

Other Components of Nutrition

Fiber

Fiber is the indigestible part of plant food. Fiber is made up of cellulose, hemicellulose, pectin and lignin. Cellulose is a carbohydrate made up of long chains of glucose. Its actual structure is slightly different from most carbohydrates however, and so amylase – the enzyme that digests carbohydrate – cannot digest cellulose. Undigested plant food (fiber) moves from the stomach into the upper intestine. Fiber has a wonderful capacity to absorb water and swell in volume. As fiber passes along the GI tract, it continues to add water and swell. This swelling allows the waste products of digestion to move more quickly and smoothly down the gut ready for elimination.

Ensuring that waste products of digestion move smoothly on their passage and exit your body in good time is absolutely essential for your health. Constipation is not only uncomfortable and sometimes embarrassing, but it can be harmful in the long term. The body's elimination system is designed to remove toxins from the body. The liver and kidneys do a great job of removing waste and toxins: the kidneys filter waste to the bladder and the liver filters toxins to the colon. When waste products hang around in the colon (large intestine) it gives much more time for toxins in the waste product to be reabsorbed into the body. If we end up "blocked up", those toxins can be reabsorbed into the body instead of being eliminated. In cultures that eat high roughage diets (twenty to thirty grams a day), there are significantly reduced incidence of diabetes, constipation and irritable bowel syndrome. Western diets that are often very low in roughage see very high incidences of these diseases.

We have to be careful however in choosing the right type of fiber to eat. Whole wheat and bran and other fiber filled cereals can certainly provide high amounts of fiber if you eat enough of them, but they also provide high amounts of carbohydrate, which is far from the goal. Ideal sources of fiber include broccoli, cauliflower, sprouted seeds and nuts, carrots, celery, lettuce, snap peas.

Some fruits are ideal sources of fiber, those with edible skins such as blueberries, apples, plums, peaches. I recall the first year I lived in my current house and the delight I experienced in summer when the golden plum tree came into fruit. Those golden plums, so yellow and ripe, were like nectar. I stood on the soft cool moss under the tree, reaching up again and again to pick a soft ripe juicy fruit from a branch. I ate plum, after plum, after plum, drinking in the juice, reveling in the rich sweet flavor that curled and rolled around my tongue and swept in waves of natural sweetness around my mouth. Less than an hour later, all that plum juice and plum fiber had a predictable effect. I now treat those plums with great respect and allocate myself a carefully calculated daily ration.

Minerals and Micronutrients

Micronutrients are nutrients required by the body in very small quantities to orchestrate a whole range of physiological functions, but which the body cannot produce itself. These are dietary minerals in amounts generally less than one hundred micrograms/day as opposed to

Micronutrient	Purpose
5HTP	Precurser to the neurotransmitter serotonin, promotes relaxed mood and sound sleep.
Alpha-GPC (L-alpha glycerylphosphorylcholine, Choline alfoscerate)	Delivers choline across the blood brain barrier and thus increases levels of the neurotransmitter acetylcholine.
Caffeine	Improves concentration, idea production, but hinders memory encoding. Also produces jitters.
Acetyl-L-carnitine (ALCAR) - Amino acid	Facilitates fatty acid utilization.
CDP-Choline (Cytidine Diphosphate Choline)	Can help improve focus and memory.
Chondroitin sulfate	Important for cartilage structure.
Coenzyme q-10 CoQ10	Helps convert food into energy and is a powerful antioxidant.
Creatine	Helps supply energy to the brain and muscles.
DMAE	Supports production of brain chemicals essential for short-term memory, concentration, and learning capacity.
Ephedrine	Increases the activity of norepinephrine – the excitatory neurotransmitter associated with stress.
Flavonoids	Potential anti-inflammatory effect.
Gamma-aminobutyric acid (GABA)	Calming neurotransmitter.
Garum armoricum extract	Adaptogen that can support stress management.
Glucosamine	Commonly used for the treatment of osteoarthritis.
Glycyrrhizic Acid	Potential anti-inflammatory effect.
Huperzine A	Potentially could improve memory skills.
Inositol	Helps the liver process fats as well as contributing to the function of muscles and nerves.
Lecithin	A source of choline.
Lipoic acid	Breaks down carbohydrates, antioxidant.
Phenibut	Helps manage anxiety.
Phosphatidylserine	Important for overall cell function.
Resveratrol	Potential antioxidant.
Theanine	An amino acid that increases serotonin and dopamine levels in the brain. Increases alpha-wave based alert relaxation.

macro-minerals which are required in larger quantities. The micro-minerals or trace elements, include but are not limited to, boron, iron, cobalt, chloride, chromium, copper, fluoride, iodine, manganese, selenium, zinc and molybdenum. Micronutrients also include vitamins which are organic compounds required in tiny amounts by the body. You can see a list of some key micronutrients and their functions in the table on the previous page.

Organic Acids

In the process of usual biological functions, the body makes a group of compounds called organic acids. It is possible to measure levels of different organic acids in urine and therefore evaluate how well certain functions are performing. Testing organic acid levels will allow a practitioner to evaluate some critical areas of metabolism including: energy production, central nervous system function, nutritional and antioxidant deficiencies, fatty acid metabolism, and to show high levels of intestinal yeast and bacteria. The right balance is important, for example, organic acids such as acetic acid and citric acid are important micronutrients.

Refined Carbohydrates

Foods which have been processed by machinery that strips the bran and germ from the whole grain are refined. The refining process gives foods a finer texture and prolongs shelf life, but it also removes important enzymes, minerals and nutrients such as B vitamins, fiber, iron and more. Sugar beet, sugar cane, wheat and rice are the basis of many foods in developed countries and all are plants that are regularly refined. The resulting food has very little nutritional value. Not only that, the refining process has reduced the chemical structure of the food such that these refined carbohydrates are very easily digested into glucose. Chemically speaking – eating white pasta or white bread is quite similar to eating candy. This type of food has lots of "almost sugar" and very little nutritional value, so anyone eating a diet composed of this type of food risks becoming malnourished in terms of nutrients.

Micronutrient Deficiencies in Crops

Vitamin and mineral supplement use is growing, partly because people want to live optimally healthy lives, partly because their diet is less than ideal, and partly because food quality is being reduced. Micronutrient deficiency in crops is widespread – an estimated fifty percent of world cereal soils are deficient in zinc, and thirty percent of cultivated soils globally are deficient in iron. Steady growth of crop yields during recent decades (in particular through the Green Revolution) compounded the problem by progressively depleting the stores of micronutrients in soil.

In general, farmers only apply micronutrients when crops show deficiency symptoms, however, micronutrient deficiencies decrease yields before symptoms appear. Some common farming practices (such as liming acid soils) contribute to widespread occurrence of micronutrient deficiencies in crops by decreasing the availability of the micronutrients present in the soil. Also, extensive use of glyphosate as a weed killer is increasingly suspected to reduce micronutrient uptake by crops, especially with regard to manganese, iron and zinc.

Vitamins

The vitamin and supplements industry is huge, HUGE, thriving even in economic downturns. Currently the vitamin and supplement industry generates $25 BILLION in sales annually. Everyone knows that vitamins are important, so there is no need to spend too much time on vitamins in this chapter. There are however some important points to note. Not all vitamin supplements are made equal. Quality varies significantly, and so do doses, so it is vital that you ask your healthcare practitioner which supplement brands they recommend. It's also important to understand that supplement and vitamin solutions that work for your friends might not be the right combination for you. There can be some excellent over-the-counter products, but your practitioner will have good ideas on which are the reliable vitamin and supplement products in combinations that are best for your particular situation, and at clinical dosing levels that will truly support an improvement in your health.

The Way Forward

It can be overwhelming working out what you need to eat more of (fresh organic vegetables, lean meat) and what you need to eat less of (refined carbohydrates), and even more overwhelming working out what vitamins, minerals and organic acids are missing from your diet. This is where your practitioner can help. If you have been eating a diet high in refined carbohydrates and low in fresh vegetables, it might be a good idea to do some micronutrient testing and/or organic acid testing. There is growing scientific evidence confirming that vitamin and mineral deficiencies are associated with the disease process. Vitamin, mineral and antioxidant deficiencies have been shown to factor in suppressed immune function and contribute to chronic degenerative processes such as arthritis, cancer, Alzheimer's, cardiovascular disease and diabetes.

Micronutrient tests measure how micronutrients are actually functioning within your white blood cells. The results give your healthcare practitioner an assessment of risk for a broad range of clinical conditions such as arthritis, cancer, cardiovascular risk, diabetes, some immune disorders, metabolic disorders and micronutrient deficiencies. There is a list in the appendix showing what labs are available to do different types of testing. Your practitioner may well be familiar with these labs and can order the testing if it is considered a good idea.

Water in the Diet

After oxygen, water is the highest priority for attaining optimum health. Why? It is quite simple – the body is over seventy percent water. The brain is over eighty-five percent water. So it makes sense that it is hard to drink too much water – pure water. The brain is the highest maintenance organ in the body and the one which controls all physiological functions, and it is the most devastated by dehydration. Staying hydrated is absolutely crucial for optimum brain function and optimum health. In fact, the number one cause of memory loss, at any age, is dehydration. Whenever you have a "senior moment", it could well be your brain telling you that your water stores are low, that you need to immediately chug a glass of pure water. Adequate hydration is not only essential for optimum brain function, it also:

- Maintains your body temperature
- Aids in digestion
- Metabolizes fat
- Lubricates and cushions your organs
- Transports nutrients throughout your body
- Flushes toxic waste from your body
- Keeps you looking and feeling young

So how much fluid is ideal per day? Many practitioners will recommend six to eight eight-ounce glasses of water or other fluids, or half of the body weight in ounces, each day as part of a healthy diet. The amount of fluids needed by the body increases with activity and as the weather gets warmer and more humid. More fluids may be helpful with a fever, congestion from a cold or cough, or other medical conditions. Some health problems require that fluid intake be limited. It is important to know how specific diseases affect fluid intake. Discuss the daily amount of fluid you need with your healthcare practitioner if you have a diagnosed health problem.

Soda, juice, milk, alcohol, tea and coffee are not good sources of water. Caffeine and alcohol are diuretics and will "pull" water from the cells in your body and eliminate it. Although it is tempting, on a hot day, to pull a cold beer or two from the fridge to quench your thirst, know that if you do that, you will need to drink twice that amount in water to rehydrate your body. For many people, the day doesn't start without a good cup of coffee. The same rule applies as to the cold beer. You will need to drink more water to make up for the impact of the caffeine. Drinking fluids other than water, soft drinks and alcohol in particular, can contribute to an intake of caloric nutrients in excess of requirements with weight gain as a result.

A (Very) Short History of Food

Going back in time again to human primitive roots, the body evolved by eating nutrient loaded foods rich in protein, essential fats, vitamins, fiber and minerals. It wasn't until the beginning of agriculture, only ten thousand years ago, that humans began to eat complex carbohydrates in significant amounts. Even then, early preparation of grain by hand was hard work, and it was prepared carefully before use.

- Grains were sprouted, which locked in B Vitamins
- Sprouting and soaking neutralized phytic acid and enzyme inhibitors in grain, essential for ensuring nutrients were available to be "used" when eaten.

It is only in the last two *hundred* years that refined sugars and refined flours began to be widely available. That is not enough time for the body to evolve new mechanisms for survival or to regulate the natural drive to "EAT SUGAR."

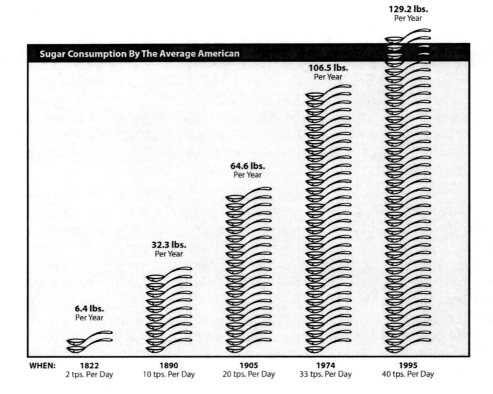

	129.2 lbs. Per Year

Sugar Consumption By The Average American

106.5 lbs. Per Year

64.6 lbs. Per Year

32.3 lbs. Per Year

6.4 lbs. Per Year

WHEN:	1822	1890	1905	1974	1995
	2 tps. Per Day	10 tps. Per Day	20 tps. Per Day	33 tps. Per Day	40 tps. Per Day

When we look at modern diets today many people eat a diet that is: high in carbohydrates, (especially refined carbohydrates); low in fiber; and loaded with trans-fats. The food quality is often poor, with inadequate amounts of micronutrients, and increasing numbers of crops are genetically modified. In addition, overeating is common due, in part, to the high amount of refined carbohydrate in many diets. The body has satiety mechanisms to tell us when we are full and have eaten enough. When we overeat on meat and unrefined carbohydrates the stomach feels full; however, refined carbohydrates have lots of calories but little fiber and nutrients and it is therefore easy to eat more than enough in a very short space of time. Most people know, but might want to not admit to, the experience of eating a whole bag of chips (eight servings at ninety calories a serving), or a gallon tub of ice cream, and yet still feeling hungry afterwards.

So what impact has this had on health? Well, chronic disease is on the rise and the numbers are staggering. This data has cropped up in the news many times in recent years, but it is worth repeating in light of the information you have just read. The data comes from the Centers for Disease Control website:

- Seven out of ten deaths among Americans each year are from chronic diseases. Heart disease, cancer, and stroke account for more than fifty percent of all deaths each year.

- In 2005, 133 million Americans – almost one out of every two adults – have at least one chronic illness.

- Obesity has become a major health concern. One in every three adults is obese, and almost one in five youths between the ages of six and nineteen is obese (BMI ≥ 95th percentile of the CDC growth chart).

- About one-fourth of people with chronic conditions have one or more daily activity limitations.

- Arthritis is the most common cause of disability, with nearly nineteen million Americans reporting activity limitations.

- Diabetes continues to be the leading cause of kidney failure, nontraumatic lower-extremity amputations, and blindness among adults aged twenty to seventy-four.

Gut Health and Gut Dysbiosis.

The "gut," or gastrointestinal system, simply refers to the long hollow tube that stretches from the tip of your tongue right down to your rectum for a whopping thirty feet. The gut is an amazing organ. About eighty percent of the body's immune system is out in full force in the gut. We take in so much stuff through the mouth that the gut has evolved to be a protector and defender in the immune system. It has hundreds of species of microbes and bacteria in there designed to help digest, serve, and protect. There are estimated to be one hundred billion (yes, billion) bacterial cells in a square millimeter of the large intestine.

Our strains of bacteria tend to develop in response to the needed defenses in the environment in which we live. If we live in the Pacific Northwest of the United States of America – it is less likely we will need to have "good" bacteria developed ready for the "bad" bacteria that lurk among vegetables in Papua New Guinea. However, if we were to travel to Papua New Guinea and be exposed to all sorts of new bacteria, chances are high that the first few days would be quite uncomfortable while the body hustled to find the right defense bacteria against the new invaders.

Microbes are not only important as front line defenders, they are also important in the digestive process, helping to metabolize nutrients so that we can absorb them more readily. In addition, the microbes and bacteria play a critical role in helping the lining of the gut replace itself. The onslaught of toxins, mixed with the digestive acids in the gut, mean the gut lining is constantly in the process of regenerating. Microbial messages are essential for making sure the replacement cells mature and migrate to the right place inside the gut. A further, and also critically important role of gut bacteria, is in the management of the immune response. Sometimes stray harmless proteins end up in the gut and there is a species of bacteria with the specific role to make sure that the immune system ignores these harmless proteins. However, if the immune cells do react to these proteins and set up a panic party, inflammation can occur, which is bad news indeed for the body.

Like any system – stability is the key for long term success. As long as the dangerous microbes coming in are defended successfully by the microbes sitting waiting to defend, then everything is fine. Think of soldiers on the battlements of a ninth century European castle ready to deal with any stray marauders. They can pick off the stray villains as long as there are not too many of them.

The bacteria in the gut are also likely to compete among themselves so that no one strain dominates over the other, thus having a plentiful supply of a variety of bacteria to defend against all sorts of incoming bacteria. When you work with a practitioner for any health related issue, it is quite likely that you will be directed to use probiotics to help support and bolster healthy gut function. Not all probiotic supplements are made equal, and your practitioner will have some recommendations for really good value probiotics.

As we know, sleep is essential for many functions, and here is another one: "bad" bacteria accumulate over the course of the day; it is when we sleep that the body works to redress the balance – to reduce the harmful bacteria to manageable levels. During the silent, dark hours of night, the melatonin surge initiates white blood cell activity specifically designed to deal with the pathogens like the "bad" bacteria living in the gut. Sleep allows the body to keep gut bacteria in balance. Lack of sleep can end up seriously messing with the system.

Normally, the gut is inhabited by trillions of good bacteria, the ones that help digest food, produce energy, and make important biological chemicals like the neurotransmitters serotonin and dopamine. When the gut is dysbiotic, this means that the "bad germs" (disease causing bacteria, for instance) begin to edge out the "good germs." When this happens, basic biological functions (such as digestion) begin to breakdown, and symptoms (stomach ache, diarrhea or constipation) begin to appear. Not all symptoms of gut dysbiosis are obvious. Because gut dysbiosis can lead to any number of physiological problems throughout the body, it can be responsible for symptoms as varied as depression to asthmatic wheezing.

When a body is unable to effectively combat the bad germs in the gut (or elsewhere in the body) the immune system can be disrupted. Hence, immune dysregulation and gut dysbiosis often occur simultaneously, and each can happen as a result of the other. Additionally, gut dysbiosis and immune dysregulation can both lead to mitochondrial dysfunction, a condition where the body's energy production is affected at the cellular level. Gut dysbiosis can therefore result in symptoms associated with mitochondrial dysfunction such as fatigue, low muscle tone, failure to thrive, motor delays and other complex health problems. It is beyond the scope of this chapter to explain in detail the function of the digestive system, but a good book that will help you understand more is "Restoring Your Digestive Health" by Jordan Rubin NMD and Joseph Brasco MD.

Symptoms of Gut Dysbiosis can include:

Symptoms of Gut Dysbiosis	
Food Intolerance	Being Underweight
Chronic Fatigue	Inflammation of the Digestive Tract
Sinus Infection	Sore Throats
PMS	Chest Problems
Food Cravings	Allergies
Ear Infections	Skin Problems
Yeast and Other Vaginal Infections	Muscle and Joint Pain
Chronic Cystitis	Nail-Bed Infections
Fluid Retention	Obesity
Hormonal Imbalance	Athlete's Foot

If you are experiencing any of these symptoms – and many people do, it is time to talk with a Functional Medicine practitioner. In addition to the micronutrient testing mentioned earlier, are other tests that your practitioner may want to order to identify what may be going on. This could include a comprehensive digestive stool analysis which looks at a number of markers to help identify and treat gastrointestinal diseases. Testing includes evaluating the following:

- Intestinal function: tests for fecal color, mucus, blood and imbalanced intestinal flora.
- Intestinal environment: tests for friendly and unfriendly bacteria as well as yeasts.
- Absorption: tests for cholesterol and fatty acids.
- Digestion: tests for triglycerides, undigested meat, fibers, pH.

Food allergies and intolerances

There are some common foods that can cause sensitivities leading to common symptoms such as migraine headaches and gut discomfort.

Most Common Food Triggers		
Dairy Products	Meat	Onions
Chocolate	Wheat/Gluten	Corn
Eggs	Nuts and Peanuts	Apples
Citrus Fruits	Tomatoes	Bananas
Red Wine	Caffeinated Drinks	Monosodium Glutamate
Aspertame	Nitrites	Sulphites

For many people, the concept that a body can be allergic to food seems just weird. The body needs food to survive, so how can foods create an allergic response? Some food allergies are well known: we hear about the anaphylactic shock that some people experience when they eat peanuts or shell fish. The reaction is swift and can be deadly as the body mounts a rapid response to a dangerous invader. These are Type 1 Food Allergies and are relatively rare – about two percent of the population experience some sort of reaction like this.

Less dramatic but also well-known are allergies to dairy products, with symptoms of gastric upset and cramps. Other food allergies have a more subtle, much less pronounced set of symptoms which can, in fact, seem so inconsequential that unless someone knows to look for the picture, it won't be visible. Understanding the full picture is a bit like trying to do a hundred piece jigsaw with only eighteen pieces. A trained healthcare practitioner skilled in understanding Functional Medicine, can take those eighteen pieces and have a better sense of what the overall picture may be. These delayed response allergic responses are known as Type 3 Allergies and are more common, although there are no clear numbers available because many cases of Type 3 food allergy are undiagnosed.

Attack and the Immune Response – some players in the game:

1. The body has a group of immune cells called Mast cells. These cells are found in the digestive tract, airways, urinary tract and in the skin cells. The job of the mast cells is to protect the body, and they have both antibacterial and antiparasitic functions.

2. Immunoglobulin antibodies are a type of molecule made instantly in response to any substance or organism that causes an immune response. Immunoglobulins are made up of chains of amino acids.

3. Antigens are any substance that, when introduced to the body, stimulates the production of antibodies.

4. An antibody is a protein produced by the body's immune system when it detects harmful substances, called antigens.

What happens in that dramatic Type 1 Food Allergy response?

Situation: a person allergic to peanuts eats a chocolate chip cookie from a plate that had peanuts on it.

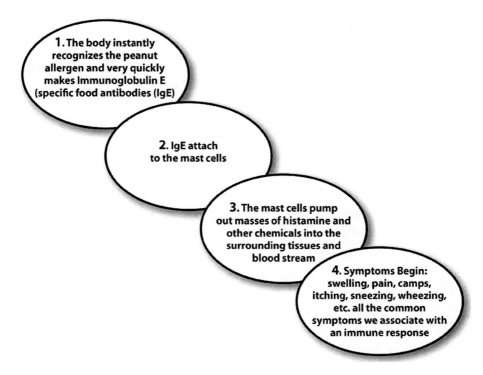

1. The body instantly recognizes the peanut allergen and very quickly makes Immunoglobulin E (specific food antibodies (IgE)

2. IgE attach to the mast cells

3. The mast cells pump out masses of histamine and other chemicals into the surrounding tissues and blood stream

4. Symptoms Begin: swelling, pain, camps, itching, sneezing, wheezing, etc. all the common symptoms we associate with an immune response

Leaky Gut

The gut is lined with mucus which contains millions of antibodies as the first line of defense against foreign bodies, and its role is to identify and neutralize anything it detects as harmful. The gut lining has more immune cells and more antibodies than any other organ in the body. A second, yet equally critical function of the mucus lining is to allow essential minerals, amino acids, essential fatty acids and other nutrients into the blood stream. Problems start to happen when this essential lining begins to break down. Where "gaps" in the lining appear, the gut now leaks bigger toxins into the blood stream. When these toxins start circulating in the body, then other antibodies are rapidly made to start clearing those toxins out. This flood of antibodies rushing around the body to sort out invaders begins the process of inflammation. At the affected places, blood flow increases and white blood cells rush in. Swelling, pain, and tenderness in these areas is the result.

For example, think of this situation. You open your back door one day and in rushes a stray dog absolutely riddled with fleas. The dog sits on the chairs, the fleas jump off; the dog sits on the carpets, the fleas jump off; the dog sits on the beds, the fleas jump off; the dog burrows in the towel closet and the fleas jump off. Now, not only do you have to get the dog out of the house, you have to clean up and de-flea all the areas the dog ran to. The house is all a flurry of rapid response action on clean up. You take on the towel closet, your daughter is dispatched to the furniture, your son is sent to clean up the beds, your spouse sets off to work on the carpets. And it takes time to settle everything back down.

When toxins find holes in the mucus lining of the gut and enter the body, just like the dog running amuck in the house, these toxins spread out to areas in the body such as joints, the heart, the kidney, or muscles. These toxins don't belong there, so antibodies have to be dispatched to clean up the toxins in different parts of the body. The rush of blood and antibodies causes swelling in the affected areas.

Okay – so now imagine that several of your doors and windows are open and the stray dog has sent the word through the neighborhood, and before long you have a pack of stray dogs jumping in through the windows and doors all spreading their fleas wherever they go. You and your family are going to spend all your time running backwards and forwards on clean up. While the doors and window are open this is going to keep happening. Soon all your energy is being spent on clean up. The same thing happens when there are multiple "holes" in the gut. Multiple toxins can get through and then travel though the blood stream to spread out through the body. The antibodies move into overdrive, constantly fighting invading toxins and increasing swelling and discomfort. Toxins in this case are the pieces of undigested food that make it through the gaps in the mucosal lining.

You may find ways to clean up the flea infested areas of your house, but as long as the doors and windows are open, those neighborhood dogs are going to keep getting in. The first thing you have to do is close up all the ways the animals are getting inside, then you have the long job of cleanup. After that, you have to make sure that those dogs do not come back into the house. (No offense is intended to the canine species with this illustration).

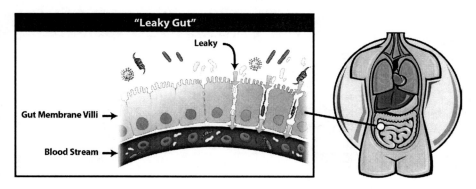

The same is true for the body. When there are holes in the mucosal lining of the gut, the first task is to begin to heal and repair those holes. As long as those holes exist, there will be a constant leakage of toxins (undigested food particles) into the body. Once the leaking gut has been healed, the next work is to heal the inflammation in different parts of the body. The next Chapter on Pain has more information on the inflammatory process.

If the gut has got to the point where it leaks constantly – there is some hard work ahead. There are some tough decisions to be made on choice of foods, and there are some choices to be made about the use of medications.

There are now a number of excellent books and internet resources to help you learn about medical interventions and about how to remove foods from your diet to see if they truly do have a harmful impact on you. Your practitioner is the best person to help you sort through your options and help formulate a plan for restoring your gut health.

There are some tests that your practitioner will probably want to do. For Type 1 Allergies – skin tests are the simple and inexpensive method. For Type 3 Delayed Food Allergy testing (food intolerances/sensitivities), then an elimination diet can be a good way to go. It can however be very time consuming and hard to take out everything without knowing where to target your attention. Blood testing can be an excellent starting point to identify possible food allergens.

To understand how blood testing for food intolerances works, we look again at Immunoglobulins. When large molecules of incompletely digested food pass through a leaking gut lining and into the blood stream, a group of antibodies called immunoglobulin–G antibodies (Ig-G) will be produced. IgG antibodies bind to the allergens that they find. A group of cells called macrophages are designed to come along and clear out the clusters of allergens/IgGs.

If these clusters are not cleared and eliminated by the macrophages, they get deposited in various vulnerable sites in the body. The blood test works by measuring IgG levels for different types of food. If a particular food type causes an immune response there will be higher levels of IgG. A test report shows which, if any, foods have spiked an immune response. Blood testing for food insensitivities does carry some risk of false positives and false negative results, however it can be a very useful starting point to work out what foods to eliminate first.

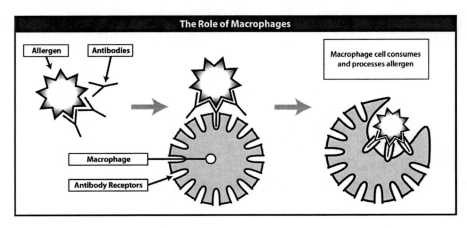

Causes of Leaky Gut

There are many factors that contribute to the development of a leaky gut or which seem to go hand in hand with the condition.

Cause	What's Happening
Hypochlorhydria	Hypochlorhydria refers to a deficiency in hydrochloric acid produced by the stomach, which can result in the body inadequately being able to assimilate foods and can lead to malnutrition.
Candidiasis	Candidiasis is a fungal infection produced by a species of Candida Fungi, particularly Candida Albicans. Candida fungi normally reside harmlessly in various parts of the body. If the healthy bacteria in the digestive tract becomes seriously depleted the candida proliferate and can produce root like structures which damage the villi along the intestinal tract leading to a 'leaky gut'. There are many causes of candidiasis such as: repeated antibiotic use, poor diet, steroid medications, birth control pills, malnutrition, cytotoxic drugs.
Dysbiosis	Dysbiosis refers to a bacterial imbalance in the gut, which can compromise the immune system.
Alcohol	Alcohol in excess is said to affect almost every organ system in the body. Alcohol increases stomach acid, contributes to hypochlorhydria and can contribute to a leaky gut. Alcohol can also cause malnutrition.
Allergies (including food)	An allergy is an abnormal reaction by our immune system to bodily contact with foreign substances that would normally be harmless.
Poor diet	Processed, packaged and convenience foods are low in nutrients and fiber and often have high levels of additives, preservatives, dyes, sugar, trans fatty acids, artificial sweeteners and other ingredients, which are considered to be harmful and have been linked with various conditions, including leaky gut.
Stress	Chronic stress can cause an inflammatory response within the body and weaken the immune system.
Parasites	Parasites are organisms that grow, feed and take shelter upon another organism whilst contributing nothing to the survival of the host. When they inhabit the gut they produce toxins and siphon off nutrients from the body.
Pharmaceuticals	NSAIDS (Non-Steroidal Anti Inflammatory Drugs) are pain relief medications that are said to increase intestinal permeability by damaging the villi in the intestine and blocking prostaglandins that stimulate tissue repair. Steroids are said to suppress the immune system, kill 'friendly' bacteria, cause the proliferation of fungal infections in the gut, all of which contribute to the development of a leaky gut. Cytotoxic drugs can certainly kill bad cells but they can also destroy good cells.

Testing for Leaky Gut

Lactulose/Mannitol Challenge Test

The Lactulose/Mannitol Challenge Test is the most common form of testing for leaky gut. Lactulose and mannitol are two water soluble, non-metabolized sugar molecules which means the full amount absorbed will be excreted. Mannitol is easily absorbed into cells, whilst lactulose has larger molecules and is only partially absorbed. After swallowing a solution containing mannitol and lactulose, urine is collected for six hours and then tested. If the levels of mannitol and lactulose in the collected urine sample are both high, it is indicative of Leaky Gut Syndrome because even the large molecules were absorbed. Low levels of both molecules indicate malabsorption of nutrients because even the small molecules were not absorbed. High levels of mannitol and low levels of lactulose indicates healthy digestion because the small molecules get in, but the big ones don't. The ratio of lactulose/mannitol is supposed to be 0.03.

Digestive Stool Analysis

This test involves testing a stool sample for: digestive function; how well fats, proteins, carbohydrates and other nutrients are absorbed in the colon; presence of candida or other bacterial infections; dysbiosis (imbalance in intestinal bacteria); parasitic infection; and other indicators of digestive dysfunction.

Candida Testing

The tests most commonly used involved testing the blood for high levels of antibodies such as IgG, IgA and IgM, which could indicate Candidiasis.

Allergy Intolerance/ Sensitivity Testing

Your practitioner can refer you for allergy testing. The methods below are the most common forms of testing that are offered:

1. A skin prick or scratch test, where a drop of fluid containing the allergen is placed on the surface of the skin and then the skin is pricked to push the allergen just under the skin surface (usually the forearm, back or upper arm). Allergies will be indicated if the skin swells, becomes itchy and red, and if a white swelling called a wheal develops, which fades after several hours. A similar test is to inject the allergen underneath the skin surface and monitor for a reaction.

2. A blood RAST (radioallergosorbent) test that measures the amount of IgE in the blood when exposed to various allergens is also used for true allergies.

3. Patch tests are used to diagnose delayed allergic reactions that cause skin rashes, such as dermatitis. Traces of the allergen are taped to the skin for forty eight hours and a dermatologist measures reactions. Tests can be performed for respiratory or food allergies.

Amino Acid Analysis

Amino acids combine to form protein required by the body. A low protein diet and poor health can cause deficiencies in amino acids. The amino acid test calculates amino acid levels in a twenty four hour urine sample. The test is used to assess the risk of heart disease; anxiety; autism; behavioral disorders; chronic fatigue; fibromyalgia; digestive disorders; along with other conditions.

Celiac Disease and Gluten Intolerance

Gluten is a protein substance found in wheat, rye, barley, oats, triticale, spelt, and kamut. Celiac disease, also known as gluten intolerance, is a genetic disorder that affects at least one in one hundred and thirty three Americans. Symptoms of celiac disease can range from mild weakness, bone pain, and mouth ulcers, to chronic diarrhea, abdominal bloating, and progressive weight loss. Gluten intolerance causes damage to the intestinal villi (the tiny fingers in the intestines needed to soak up nutrients from food). When someone with celiac disease eats gluten, the lining of their small intestine becomes inflamed and damaged, which hampers the absorption of nutrients and can lead to malnutrition and weight loss.

If someone with true celiac disease continues to eat gluten, studies have shown that he or she will increase their chances of gastrointestinal cancer by a factor of forty to one hundred times that of the normal population. Further, gastrointestinal carcinoma or lymphoma develops in up to fifteen percent of patients with untreated celiac disease. It is therefore really important that the disease is quickly and properly diagnosed so it can be treated as soon as possible.

Diagnosing Gluten Intolerance/Celiac Disease

Blood testing is a good starting point to establish if IgG levels are high. Eliminating gluten from the diet for six weeks and then reintroducing is a good way to evaluate the impact of gluten on the body. An endoscopy is another procedure to confirm diagnosis. An endoscopy is an examination and biopsy of the tissue of the small intestine, often used to test for celiac disease (as well as several other non-food-related conditions). In this test, a flexible tube with a camera attached is lowered into the stomach, usually through the esophagus. When checking for celiac disease, gastroenterologists look for patterns of damage in the villi and, with celiac disease, the villi are likely to be flat.

Gluten Sensitivity

Gluten can set off a distinct reaction in the intestines and the immune system even in people who do not have celiac disease. The symptoms are often the same as celiac disease although generally not as severe, and an endoscopy usually reveals that the villi usually are not flattened. Recent research has looked at lots of different bio-markers and concluded that celiac disease and gluten sensitivity are two separate diseases, brought on by different immune responses in the body, even though they have similar symptoms.

To people who experience the symptoms, knowing there is a technical difference between celiac disease and gluten sensitivity can be like splitting hairs, they have the symptoms and, when they take gluten out of their diets, they begin to feel much better. Whether someone has celiac disease or gluten sensitivity, the treatment is all the same – take gluten out of the diet. To continue to put gluten into the body is to set the body up for a constant battle that is both tiring and, in the long term, potentially dangerous.

For resources on living with gluten intolerance or gluten sensitivity go to www.celiac.com.

A Final Word

Although there are indications that diet can have some impact on a number of different types of cancer, the types of cancer that seem most strongly linked to diet are found in two groups in the body:

1. The parts of the body involved in digestion – stomach, liver, pancreas, colon.

2. Organs where estrogen plays a significant role – the breasts, ovaries, uterus, and, in men, the prostate. A high animal fat diet can significantly increase the amount of estrogen that the body makes, and higher levels of estrogen carry the risks associated with estrogen dominance including elevated risks of developing cancer.

Whether you have a history of cancer in your family, or are currently working to heal the disease, lifestyle factors, including your diet, can make a huge difference in helping you defend against cancer. Some foods actually increase your risk of cancer, while others support your body and strengthen your immune system. By making smart nutrition choices, you can protect your health, feel better, and boost your ability to fight off cancer and other diseases.

Using the information in this chapter on the basics of how nutrition works in the body, you can now ask your practitioner for recommendations on treatment and nutrition choices. You could probably make some good strides on your own by changing the choices you make about food, and yet, if you are experiencing chronic symptoms, it is likely that you will need the help of a Functional Medicine professional who can diagnose the root cause of dis-ease and then develop a treatment plan that is right for you. With the information you now have, you will have a deeper understanding of the testing and treatment recommendations your practitioner will choose.

Chapter Three Summary – Nutrition

- The major components of food: protein, carbohydrate and fats
- Other food components: fiber, micronutrients, organic acids, vitamins, hydration
- Changes in food quality and consumption
- Gut health and dysbiosis
- Leaky gut
- Food allergies
- Testing nutritional status

CHAPTER FOUR

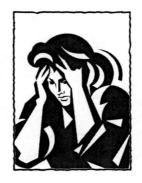

PAIN

Sitting at my kitchen counter one cold winter afternoon, working with my wood carving tools, a momentary lapse of concentration resulted in a three quarter inch cut as a very sharp steel gouge pierced the fleshy pad on my left thumb. My brain registered the knowledge of the incident before it experienced the pain of it. As adrenaline began to surge into my brain I rushed to the sink, held my hand over the bowl, a clean piece of paper towel clamped over the two sides of the wound, my brain working in two parts. The problem solving part of my brain, reinforced by the adrenaline surge, was saying "clamp the wound shut, apply pressure, elevate your hand, focus". Another part of my brain was saying *"Ow, Ow, Ow, Ow"*.

The Ow's took a back seat as endorphins kicked in to act as a short term painkiller, thus allowing my thinking brain to take the lead and evaluate the situation. Had the blood clotted yet? Had I severed a major blood vessel? Would I need stiches? Should I go to Emergency? Is there any wood in the wound? What's the best way to clean this? My brain was evaluating the situation and taking action, then, with the understanding that it was not life threatening, the stinging *OW, OW, OW, OW,* message got louder.

With a bandage in place, my brain started to calm down and I could begin to take some deep breaths and move on from life preserving problem solving. As the adrenaline level dropped, my breathing rate slowed and became deeper. The OW's had it at the stage, and they were shouting loud. As this was happening I was fascinated to think through the biochemistry of my thumb's unexpected encounter with the very sharp business end of a wood carving gouge.

Recent studies of pain mechanisms have discovered receptors in the skin that send pain information to the Central Nervous System (CNS). In most cases the initial stimulus for pain is the destruction or injury of tissue next to certain nerve fibers; in my case, the point at which the gouge went sharply through my skin and into the flesh.

For very practical survival purposes, the CNS has evolved special pathways to send pain and temperature information to the brain to ensure that a quick response happens when there is damage to the body. Pain messages are transmitted to the brain via two specific pathways called delta fibers and c-fibers. Receptors that respond to noxious (harmful/toxic/injurious) stimulation are called nociceptors (nerve endings). Nociceptors are activated by pain, and they transmit extremely fast electrical signals through the delta fibers to the spinal cord whereby the message goes swiftly up the spinal cord to the brain. Nociceptors have a second job, they trigger chemical messenger release signals which travel "slower" along the c-fibers into the spinal cord and on to the brain. The chemicals released include neuropeptides, serotonin, histamine, some enzymes, prostaglandins (a group of widespread hormones), endorphins, and nerve growth factor. These messengers are received in different parts of the brain but collectively they mount the response to the painful stimulus. The nervous system gets the signal to regulate breathing, blood flow, pulse rate, the feeling of pain, and to release cortisol and adrenaline.

Skin is a vital organ, it is the absolutely essential wrapping that keeps everything in the body in place and secure. The loss of skin mass immediately threatens the life of the individual through blood loss and potential infection. Skin is like the defensive walls that run around a medieval castle. Just as the castle walls are essential for keeping out marauders, intact skin is of vital importance to protect the body against the environment; any breach in the defenses immediately activates mechanisms to repair the opening. A skin wound is any loss of skin integrity: a cut, a graze, an insect sting, a splinter, a blister, a burn, a rash. Such a loss can result suddenly, either from fire or mechanical accident (such as a wood carving gouge), or it can occur in a chronic manner due to illness, as in skin ulcers. Skin wound healing is a dynamic biological process that begins with tissue injury. It has several goals:

1. Stop any further injury.

2. Repair injured cells.

3. Form new tissue.

4. Make the new tissue to be very like the pre-injury skin in terms of form and function.

These events have traditionally been divided into three overlapping phases: an inflammatory phase, a proliferative phase, and a maturation phase. Any time there is damage to the skin, the repair response will swing into action. The body is truly incredible in its capacity to heal damage.

The inflammatory phase is the first response to the injury. Blood vessels have usually been cut and there is bleeding. Because blood is the vital fluid in the body, the first order of the day is for the body to stop the leakage of blood as fast as possible. A blood clot is the mechanism the body has developed, a naturally produced blockage that stops up the damaged blood vessel. This is what I was watching for as I held my wound tightly while I waited for the blood clotting process to get underway. The body also constricts blood vessels at this point, reducing the flow of blood into the area and thus limiting further the potential loss of blood. I did notice that my left hand looked white, as if there was less blood in the area.

After several minutes however, once the clotting process is working and the breach in the skin is filled with blood clots, the acute inflammatory response then begins. C-fibers interact with wounds by signaling the need for repair. A range of chemical messengers called pro-inflammatory cytokines, neutrophils, and macrophages signal the need for protection against infection and the promotion of healing. These signals tell the body to allow blood to flow back into the area around the wound. White blood cells (leucocytes) arrive in the blood stream to defend the body against foreign debris and bacteria. White blood cells also release growth factors to start the healing process and grow new cells and skin. The c-fibers continue to send messages of pain so that the affected area is painful and thus (hopefully) left to rest. After bandaging my wound, there was nothing much left for me to do but to respect the pain in my thumb, recline gracefully on the sofa with my arm elevated, and watch a movie. Truly, it was a medical necessity.

Over the next few days, my wound continued to heal itself. This was the proliferative stage of wound healing. The two sides of the cut began to reconnect, tissue was rebuilt, blood vessels rejoined, white blood cells continued their patrol against possible invaders, the bruising declined, and gradually the swelling went down. I had to be careful though, as there was still significant pain in my thumb. Some motions were fine, I could grasp a wine glass (thank goodness), and type these words, but other actions created either a stabbing sharp burst of pain at the wound site or a pounding throbbing ache in the whole thumb. This pain was a message, a reminder that there was still significant repair activity underway and it was time for me to back off and be careful. Within a week the bandage was off and the scar tissue was beginning to get thinner and stronger. After two weeks, I had full range of motion of my thumb and the scar tissue was pale and barely noticeable. This was the maturation phase of wound healing and by now a large proportion of the healing was completed.

I was able to take good care of the wound – even if it meant I had to sit still and watch more movies and football than usual. If I had gone outside to deal with any of the multitude of yard care activities that demand attention in January – I would have risked interfering with the healing process. If I had clipped back one of the hedges, I would have risked tearing and bruising the replacement tissue. If I had caught my thumb on a blackberry thorn, opened up the scar and got bacteria in the wound, I would have risked infection. In addition, if I had a suppressed immune system (oh wait – I have), or if I had injuries of the nervous system, diabetes mellitus, atherosclerosis and other vascular diseases, metabolic and ageing problems, any of these could have affected one or more phases of wound healing. But by allowing the wound to heal, eating right and resting, it quickly returned to full health.

The body has a systematic approach for dealing with wounding: for halting further damage, repelling invaders, and repairing tissue. When the body is unable to work through this systematic approach to healing a wound, then that wound is considered to be chronic. Such chronic wounds can last for weeks, months, or even years, and, despite adequate and appropriate care, they are difficult and frustrating to manage. People with chronic wounds experience discomfort and stress, and are faced with the high cost of long-term conventional treatment required for such wounds to heal.

This chapter began by using a very real example of an injury to illustrate the role of pain and an overview of the process of healing. The pain referred to in this example is acute pain, pain that comes from a specific event, a known cause that happens and then goes away as healing is complete. Other examples of acute physical pain include:

- Bee or nettle sting.
- Impact such as banging your head on an overhead beam.
- Trapping your hand in a door frame.

- Touching a hot dish.
- Scalding yourself with hot water.
- Gunshot wound.
- Bone fracture.
- Torn muscle or tendon.

However, chronic pain is different. Chronic pain is where pain goes on abnormally long, where pain drags on for weeks, months, years. Chronic pain can be due to a persistent medical condition or disease, or from a serious infection, from misalignment of joints. It can also continue long after the initial problem, for example in the situation of phantom limb pain several months or years after an amputation. To understand the mechanisms of chronic pain and therefore what to do about it, we have to look first at the "usual" course of the healing process, and then look at where some of those mechanisms have gone wrong.

Most of us are familiar with looking at different systems in the body and that "systems thinking" is a way of understanding how complex parts all fit together. Understanding pain through a systems perspective is a powerful way to look deeply into what is going on with a specific area of chronic pain, and thus work with a practitioner to repair where the system has gone awry. Taking a systems approach to understanding chronic pain allows treatment beyond simply taking pain killers to mask symptoms, into a place of correcting what has gone wrong.

Take a moment to visualize the rooms in your home. Each room may be decorated differently and have a different specific function, or perhaps some multiple functions. There are doorways between some of the rooms of the home and not others. Your home has several separate rooms, yet there are many things that connect all the rooms together. The heating system runs throughout the home, the style of wood trim, the electrical system, the plumbing system, the framing, the exterior look and feel of the home. The home operates as a system with separate parts (rooms) interconnected.

The body has three major systems related to pain that function as separate parts and also interrelate with each other.

- Nervous System
- Endocrine System
- Immune System

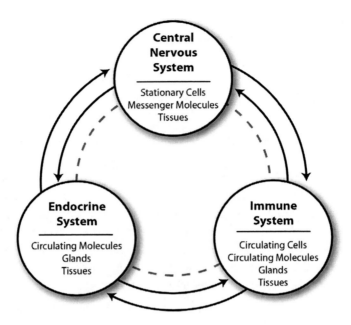

The Nervous System

A major purpose of the nervous system is to transmit information to the brain about a place of damage, so that the brain can then start a series of actions to repair the damage. The nervous system interacts directly with the immune system when the chemical messengers at the impact point call up the immune response to help create the inflammation response. The nervous system and the immune system combine to create a laundry list of chemicals necessary for immediate and longer term response. The feedback loops between the injury point and the brain continue as long as healing is in process.

The Endocrine System

The Endocrine System operates as a primary messenger system. There are two primary ways the endocrine system interacts with the nervous system in response to pain. The first is known as the defensive arousal stage. The neurotransmitter norepinephrine (noradrenaline) and epinephrine (adrenaline) are the go-betweens for the stress response to pain. The neurotransmitter acetylcholine is released from the nervous system in response to trauma, and acetylcholine triggers the secretion of norepinephrine and epinephrine. Epinephrine is produced in the part of the adrenal gland called the adrenal medulla and its purpose is to put the brain/body on alert, to heighten vigilance, attention and fear, to be ready to fight or flee or freeze. Norepinephrine and epinephrine increase heart rate and breathing, tighten muscles, constrict blood vessels in parts of the body, and initiate increased blood flow to the heart, brain, lungs and muscles.

The endocrine system is then also involved with the recovery stage. This actually begins before the defensive stage ends, which is an inbuilt mechanism designed to counterbalance the defensive stage. If the body stays on alert for too long then neurotransmitters can be depleted or the system broken. As norepinephrine and epinephrine rise, so will cortisol production. As cortisol increases in response to norepinephrine and epinephrine then a feedback mechanism created by higher levels of cortisol shuts down the production of norepinephrine and epinephrine. This allows the body to return back to a calmer state and to suppress the inflammatory response. (This is an important point to remember for the Chapter on Stress – cortisol's role on increasing and maintaining inflammation).

The Immune System

While the nervous system houses the primary mechanisms for detecting and defending against *outside* threats to the body, the immune system houses the primary mechanisms for defending what happens *inside* the body. As soon as there is any wound, any disruption to homeostasis in the body, the immune system is there at the ready. The immune system is triggered into response through several mechanisms: from blood borne messengers from the wound itself, from messages from nociceptors in the nervous system, and from the endocrine system in the form of neurotransmitters.

For a visual of this – let us return to the castle imagery. Imagine a mediaeval castle, it has a central Keep in the middle, open space around the Keep, and then a huge wall, five feet thick and thirty feet tall, built of stones, running all the way around the outside. The immune system is the big maintenance crew on the inside of the castle walls – looking out for everything that needs taking care of and doing all the repairs within the castle grounds. In addition, as soon as there is a breach of the castle walls from incoming marauders then a significant number of the immune system crew are dispatched immediately to deal with the situation. Their first purpose is to create a barrier against the attacking marauders by mounting a defense against anyone or anything trying to get in, dispatching those who do, while simultaneously working to rebuild the wall from the outside in. The castle wall will lose is smooth, seamless appearance in the short term as the flurry of activity draws lots of workers to the site.

As the repairs are completed and the marauders rebuffed, the area once again looks like it used to, apart from the "scar" where the replacement stones were put back in place and the wall rebuilt.

The same is true at any point of injury on the body: redness, pain, heat, and swelling are the usual signs related to the natural process of inflammation. Good inflammation is healing inflammation. When the repair to the damaged tissue is completed, heat declines, swelling goes down, pain reduces, and eventually all that is left is a small scar.

{ Natural Defense Mechanisms to Pain }

Estrogen • Progesterone • Prostaglandins • Endorphins
Antioxidants • Vitamin C • Vitamin E • Beta Carotene

How do all the right messages get conveyed around the body? Well, cytokines are one of the immune system's major signaling mechanisms. Cytokines are like the alarm trumpets that are blown to tell everyone in the castle that the castle is under attack. Cytokines are produced in part to signal to all the cell types needed to respond to the injury. The immune system will sense what the nervous system cannot. The immune system senses microbial invasion, toxins, tumors, and injuries to individual cells. It first evaluates (is this self or not-self?), makes decisions (what needs to happen?), takes action (inflammatory response and directing cells to the right place), and it learns from the past experience (adaptive immunity and conditioning). The signs of inflammatory response are pain, heat, swelling and redness. Inflammation reduces function and increases pain by making the nociceptors more sensitive. While this is happening, the nervous system continues to monitor the activity of the immune system.

Cytokines are a diverse group of proteins that function as signalers within and between cells. Some cytokines are proinflammatory – they cause inflammation, and some are anti-inflammatory. It is possible to evaluate someone's response to inflammation by measuring the relative numbers of proinflammatory and anti-inflammatory cytokines that are present in the blood stream. An anti-inflammatory cytokine that many people are familiar with is Insulin-like growth factor 1 (IGF-1).

When we get sick from something – a virus or bacterial infection for example, we experience a whole host of symptoms: fever, lack of energy, fatigue, difficulty concentrating, sleepiness, decreased appetite and libido, and more pain. There is also growing support for the idea that the immune response can also increase depression. This "sickness response" could be a clever adaptation to make the body slow down, and create time and space to focus on responding to the infection. When you look at it like that, you just have to stand back and be filled with awe at how the body is designed to make us rest when there is damage or infection that needs repair. The problem, of course, is when there is a permanent disease state, and permanent pain; in this situation the depressive state can go on, and on, and on, and on.

Free Radicals

Free radicals, also known as oxidants, are harmful by-products of the natural cell metabolism that occurs in the human body on a continuous basis. When there is inflammation, tissue damage etc, the body's process of clean up and repair will increase the level of free radicals in the body. Free radicals cause damage by attacking the body's tissue. If your body is sick or working on wound healing, you can help the healing process by taking extra antioxidants to knock out the free radicals. If inflammation runs unchecked for a number of years, the situation is not only painful, it can be dangerous to the body. Free radicals can attack DNA, leading to dysfunction, mutation, and possibly to cancer. Free radicals can attack enzymes and proteins, disrupting normal cell activities, or cell membranes, producing a chain reaction of destruction. Such membrane damage in the cells that line the blood vessels can lead to hardening and thickening of the arteries and eventually to heart attacks and strokes. Free-radical attacks on collagen can cause cross-linking of protein molecules, resulting in stiffness in the tissue. Free radicals are cleared out of the body by antioxidants. Well known antioxidants are: vitamin C and E, blueberries, red beans and kidney beans.

Let's take a break from this chunky biochemistry to look at some common specific pain conditions. We can take the theory we have reviewed in the first few pages of this chapter and apply it to real life situations that many people are dealing with.

Crohn's Disease

Crohn's disease is an inflammatory bowel disease, or IBD. Crohn's disease usually occurs in the small intestine (the ileum) and the large intestine (the colon), but it can happen anywhere in the digestive tract. In Crohn's disease, the immune system produces too much of a cytokine called tumor necrosis factor-alpha (TNF-alpha). TNF-alpha attacks healthy cells in the gastrointestinal (GI) tract which triggers the inflammation that leads to the painful symptoms of Crohn's disease. Typical Crohn's disease symptoms include frequent diarrhea, abdominal pain, fever, sometimes rectal bleeding, or weight loss, but may also cause complications outside the gastrointestinal tract, such as skin rashes, arthritis, inflammation of the eye, tiredness and lack of concentration. It can also lead to damage to the GI tract that may require surgery.

Crohn's disease is caused by interactions between environmental, immunological and bacterial factors in people who are genetically susceptible, and results in a chronic inflammatory disorder. Crohn's disease has traditionally been described as an autoimmune disease, but some recent investigators have begun to describe it as an immune deficiency state.

Ulcerative Colitis (UC)

UC is another form of inflammatory bowel disease. It is a form of colitis which is an inflammation of the lining of the colon, and includes ulcers, or open sores along parts or all of the colon. The main symptom of active disease is usually constant diarrhea mixed with blood, that starts gradually. IBD is often confused with irritable bowel syndrome (IBS), which is a troublesome, but much less serious, condition. Ulcerative colitis has similarities to Crohn's disease. Ulcerative colitis is an intermittent disease, with flare-ups in symptoms followed by periods that are relatively symptom-free. Although the symptoms of ulcerative colitis can sometimes diminish on their own, the disease often requires treatment with anti-inflammatory drugs such as steroids to go into remission. It can result in some nasty side effects including bloating, anemia, pain and damage to self-esteem.

The disease is more prevalent in northern countries of the world (where Vitamin D levels are often chronically low), as well as in northern areas of individual countries or other regions. Rates tend to be higher in the wealthier countries of the world. The disease may be triggered in a susceptible person by environmental factors such as food allergies, additives, emotional stress, a diet high in refined foods, intestinal parasites, or the abuse of laxatives. Those suffering from Crohn's, Colitis or UC have a significantly higher risk of colon cancer than non-sufferers and so may benefit from the preventative screening of a regular colonoscopy.

Ulcerative colitis is treated as an autoimmune disease. Standard allopathic treatment is often with anti-inflammatory drugs, immunosuppression, and biological therapy targeting specific components of the immune response. A colectomy (partial or total removal of the large bowel through surgery) is occasionally necessary, but is not a cure for the disease. In contrast, many naturopathic and Functional Medicine practitioners have great success in treating colitis through diet and lifestyle changes. Utilizing a planned sequence of changes to diet and supplements that support healthy intestinal function, it is possible to turn around colitis and restore a patient to health very effectively. A significant aspect of healing and recovering from colitis includes addressing psychological factors. Colitis is so frequently influenced by emotions that treatment frequently includes relaxation therapy, emotional work, and lifestyle changes. All activities that evoke stress, destructive emotions, or require a hurried pace, must be avoided or handled differently. Even the best treatment approach will not work when the mind and emotions are in turmoil.

Joint Pain

Over forty three million women in the US suffer from joint pain, stiffness, and the associated anxiety, stress and depression of arthritis. Rheumatoid Arthritis (RA) and Osteoarthritis (OA) together beat heart disease and stroke as the major causes of disability. OA is degenerative joint disease in which the cartilage (connective tissue between bones) breaks down so that the bones rub together causing pain. The bone can become thickened and distorted and joints no longer work with ease. The major risk factors for OA are age, injury, diet, obesity, and wearing high heeled shoes. (Sorry ladies). Carrying extra weight is a major risk factor because the extra weight puts considerable pressure on the soft connective tissue between joints. Wherever there is too much pressure, there will be pain. Whenever there is pain, the inflammatory response will be in action.

Foods that help with joint pain include: Fresh fish (not farmed) that are high in Omega 3 oils; leafy vegetables (rich in antioxidants to help destroy free radicals); flax seeds, and vitamin B3. There are also a number of herbs that can help with pain relief and inflammation - your practitioner can help you determine which are the right herbs for you.

Rheumatoid Arthritis (RA) is characterized by morning stiffness, swollen joints, stiff neck, swollen and sore wrists, fingers, ankles, toes, and difficulty bending and moving. In particular, the joint linings, bones and cartilage can all become painfully inflamed. As an RA warrior I personally understand how RA can be debilitating. I developed a variant of RA called

Ankylosing Spondylitis shortly after my second daughter was born. Starting with my right knee, followed by my left wrist, my right ankle, my left elbow, gradually all my major joints began to accumulate fluid. Within three years I struggled to open jars, bend down to play with my girls on the floor, reach for items that were always being dropped, move quickly to catch the girls, get in and out of chairs, turn to look at something without pain, hold pans without dropping them, turn the steering wheel on the car, walk. During flare ups, my body would be in such pain, and the fatigue would be so debilitating, that when I had taken my daughters to preschool – I would then sit immobile in a chair until it was time to pick them up a few hours later. Any movement I made resulted in a cascade of pain throughout my body, and I needed to save all my energy for the three hours between 3pm and 6pm while I waited for their father to arrive home and help out.

As we know, the first stage of an inflammatory response involves the body asking a question of its self – is this self or not self? In a well-functioning immune system – only the "not self" situations cause the immune response to trigger. In RA – the immune response triggers on "self" – and begins an inward defense attack. The soft tissue around joints (the synomium) is a usual place for the attack to begin. The synomium becomes inflamed, it grows more cells which then divide and grow more cells, so the synomium becomes thickened and the joint becomes swollen. The abnormal cells invade cartilage and bone and then the muscles, ligaments, and tendons surrounding the joint become weak. This leads to pain and, long term, to deformity. RA is most likely to begin between the ages of thirty and sixty and is linked to an increased risk of osteoporosis. Some interesting facts:

- RA is far more likely to impact women.
- RA is likely to be reduced during pregnancy.
- RA is likely to flare up when pregnancy is over (my case).
- RA is likely to be linked to psychological distress.

Lower Back Pain

As many as fifty percent of people in America may experience lower back pain over the course of one year. The spine functions not only as the major framework for the body, but as the main highway of the central nervous system, sending information from all regions of the body to the brain and also transmitting messages out from the brain. All lower back pain will be made worse by being overweight because the extra pounds will strain the joints further. The causes of lower back pain fall into three main groups: muscular and soft tissue, structural, and organic.

Causes of Lower Back Pain		
Muscular and Soft Tissue	**Structural**	**Organic**
Acute Muscle Strain	Disc Displacement	Infection or Disease in one of the organs of the body eg. Kidney Disease
Muscle Injury	Sciatica	
Long Term Postural Strain	Compression Fractures *Which may be associated with osteoporosis*	Cancer that spreads to the spine
Muscle Inflammation		Aneurysms
Fibromyalgia	Degeneration of the Vertebrae	
	Scoliosis	
	Genetic Abnormalities	

Osteoporosis

Osteoporosis is a metabolic bone disease. Just like any other cell in the body, bone is alive and will naturally replace itself. Most people think of bones being hard and solid, like a steel bar, however, viewed in cross section it is easy to see that bone is structured like a honey comb, with spaces in-between the hard elements. The size of the spaces depends on the person and which bone. The outer layer of bone is the hardest because it is composed of compact bone tissue, so-called due to its minimal gaps and spaces. Its porosity is 5–30%. This tissue gives bones their smooth, white and solid appearance and accounts for 80% of the total bone mass of an adult skeleton. Compact bone may also be referred to as dense bone. Filling the interior of the bone is spongy bone, which makes the overall bone lighter and allows room for blood vessels and bone marrow. Spongy bone accounts for the remaining 20% of total bone mass, but has nearly ten times the surface area of compact bone. Its porosity is 30–90%.

Bones are living parts of the body - we constantly make and lose bone. All through childhood, adolescence and early adulthood, we make more bone than we lose. After about thirty years of age there is a switch and we begin to lose more bone than we make. We are all told that calcium is needed to keep bones strong, but vitamin D, magnesium, vitamin K, and strontium are also necessary for healthy bone building, so including all in the diet is essential for giving bones the resources they need to be strong. Hormones are important for bone health too. Estrogen helps prevent reabsorption of bone, while progesterone stimulates bone building cells (osteoblasts) to build new bone. Following menopause the rate at which women lose bone increases, so ensuring optimal hormone levels helps maintain healthy bones.

A proactive step to maintaining bone strength and density is to include weight bearing exercise in weekly activities. Nowhere in the body is "use it or lose it" more relevant than in the maintenance of strong bones. In addition, replacing alcohol with vitamin water drinks, stopping smoking, and reducing caffeine intake all help to maintain bone integrity.

Because osteoporosis is a metabolic disease, it doesn't really have symptoms and so is hard to detect without a bone density scan; often the first sign of osteoporosis is a fracture from a fall that should not have caused a fracture. As osteoporosis progresses, the bones in the spine begin to collapse in on themselves, so people with osteoporosis will lose height and can developed curved spines.

In addition to bones and muscles, the body's various parts are held together and padded by tendons, ligaments, bursae and menisci.

- Tendons are fibrous chords that attach muscle to bones and they can be damaged when repeated motions cause tiny tears in the fiber.

- Ligaments are the wiry structures that connect bone to bone and keep joints stable. Damage to ligaments, e.g. twisting and tearing, can be severe enough to require surgery to reconnect the "wires".

- Bursae are the cushioning sacs of fluid that allow muscles to move smoothly over bones. Bursitis occurs when the bursa is swollen and inflamed – usually through damage or over use.

- Menisci are tough, cartilage shock absorbers inside joints and the most common sort of damage is tearing.

Inflammation is the standard response to any damage of tendons, ligaments, bursae and menisci, and the inflammation and repair of the tendon results in scar tissue and thickening of the tendon. The most common areas damaged include the major joints – knees, hips, ankles, shoulders, elbows and wrists, however repetitive strain damage can also occur in any joint. Vitamin C in high doses helps with the inflammation as it is a powerful antioxidant and chases away the free radicals that run rampant when there is tissue damage. Other tools to use include Vitamins

E, A, and B, Zinc, Selenium, Calcium and Magnesium, Omega EPA, proteolytic enzymes and curcumin. Working with a practitioner skilled in understanding the correct balance of micronutrients is vital for ensuring effective long term recovery from musculoskeletal damage.

Headaches and Migraines

Headaches are a big problem. They hurt. They debilitate. They can be so bad we wish we could just die to get away from them. They can make us sick. They make us lose days at work or time with family. Statistics from the Centers for Disease Control suggest that over one in five women, and one in ten men, regularly experience headaches that last one day or more.

Common causes of headaches include dehydration, food allergies, emotional stress, environmental toxins (perfumes, chemicals), bright lights, too little sleep, low blood sugar, eye strain, muscle damage, medications, hormone imbalances, even changes in the weather!

If you suffer from bad headaches – either tension or migraines, you may want to check your salivary hormone levels, test for un-known food allergies, make sure you eat regularly (avoid sugary snacks), improve the amount and quality of your sleep, and stay well hydrated. If your headaches are tension headaches you may want to look into Structural Deep Tissue Massage which is helpful for releasing tight muscles that create painful areas which restrict movement. A combination of damage, poor posture, and compensatory movements can result in muscle fibers fusing together. Fused muscles will then compound the problem as stressed muscles can block oxygen circulation and distribution of nutrients in the body. Deep tissue massage improves oxygen circulation and body fluid movement by breaking up and eliminating scar tissue that is found on stressed muscles. This not only allows injured muscle tissue to heal, but it also helps remove toxins such as lactic acid and cellular wastes from the system. In addition it relaxes tense muscles through kneading motions using different levels of pressure. Deep tissue massage is even used on more serious conditions and chronic diseases such as osteoporosis, fibromyalgia and carpal tunnel syndrome.

Fibromyalgia

Fibromyalgia is a multidimensional chronic pain disorder that affects approximately two percent of the population, mainly women. The common symptoms are unrefreshing sleep, muscle pain throughout the body, morning stiffness, weakness, fatigue, decreased mental clarity and problems with memory. Linked symptoms can be IBS, low blood pressure, wobbly balance, headaches, migraines, and sensitivity to bright light and loud noises. For many years fibromyalgia was often ignored and discounted by many clinicians, but in the last ten years there has been more focus to find solutions for this diagnosis. Some new ways of thinking about fibromyalgia suggest that the usual mechanisms for responding to trauma or damage get stuck in the "on" position. When stuck in the "on" position, the systemic response to pain remains active, the hormones and neurotransmitters and other molecules released to deal with trauma/injury/damage don't switch off, and a situation of permanent inflammation occurs. It is a viscous cycle at this point. Inflammation, begets inflammation, that begets inflammation.

The cycle above can begin in a number of ways:

1. Repeated injury to a particular area of the body (e.g. through over use, over training)

2. Living in a stressful environment

3. A lifestyle that causes stress to the body and mind

4. PTSD (from a range of emotionally stressful situations)

5. Inability to rest and relax from a trauma and heal

6. Wounding or surgery

7. Diseases that cause nerve damage

The Serotonin Pathway

Serotonin is one of the major neurotransmitters in the body. It plays a role in sleep, pain thresholds, blood flow, hunger/satiety, and libido. It also plays a major role in depression, anxiety, and possibly obsessive-compulsive disorders. There are now studies that indicate that supporting serotonin production – through the use of 5hydroxy-tryptophan, can cause significant improvement in anxiety, pain intensity, quality of sleep, fatigue, and the number of tender points experienced by a patient with fibromyalgia. Your practitioner will know whether to test neurotransmitters based on your symptoms, and, if your serotonin levels are low, can recommend a good supplement that has the right cofactors (including Vitamin B) to make enough of the right neurotransmitters.

Exercise

Someone with fibromyalgia probably feels more like taking a vacation in hell than taking exercise, however, anytime exercise is possible – even a twenty minute walk or fifteen minutes on a stationary bike, it will bring positive results. Exercise regulates the release of neurotransmitters, all of which have an impact on mood, energy levels and pain sensitivity. Exercise is also vital for helping ensure good blood flow throughout the body. Plaque naturally builds up on the inside of the arteries. When plaque builds up, blood flow becomes sluggish, cutting off the flow of nutrients and oxygen to other areas of the body and thus reducing the available nutrients needed for repairing general wear and tear. The more blockages there are in the body, the less flow, fewer nutrients are delivered, and so areas that have been damaged or are inflamed will take significantly longer to repair. Exercise, even mild exercise, will increase the flow of blood throughout the body thus providing nutrients and oxygen much needed for repair.

Food to help reduce inflammation

Certain foods and nutrients are vital for giving your body the tools for cleaning and repair. Pain is felt as a result of damage, for example in fibromyalgia, IBS, injured muscle/bones, ulcers etc. Remember that whenever there is pain and inflammation, free radicals are running rampant and they need to be "taken down". You need the right tools (nutrients) for that process. You wouldn't set out to clean your kitchen armed with a knife, a roll of duct tape, a pair of bunny slippers and a pint of engine oil, you would get a sponge, detergent, the vacuum, and plenty of water.

Your major tools for reducing inflammation are antioxidants. Vitamins C and E are vital, as is beta carotene. Beta carotene is found on the cell membrane and helps protect a cell from any free radicals that approach. The chart on the next page shows a list of Inflammatory Foods and Anti-inflammatory Foods.

Inflammatory Foods	Anti-Inflammatory Foods
Animal Fats	Fresh caught cold water fish (Omega 3 oils)
Alcohol	Brown rice
Citrus Fruits	Cooked or dried fruits
High Allergen foods: wheat, oats, gluten, dairy, nuts, eggs, corn	Cooked green, yellow, orange and red vegetables – broccoli, Brussels, chard, greens
Potatoes	Spinach
Lard	Squash
Butter	Sweet potatoes including taro (poi)
Excess Salt	Water
Sulphites	Condiments
Tomatoes	Green tea
Corn Oil (esp GMO)	Blueberries and blackcurrants
High fructose corn syrup	Alpha lipoic acid in vegetables, beans and fruits
Any Farmed fish (fed on soy beans, high in Omega 6 and overcrowded, so sick)	Flax seed oil, walnut oil, coconut oil
Diet Soda	Oat products (unless gluten intolerant)
	Curcumin
	Glutathione

In addition to antioxidants – here are some other ideas your practitioner may consider in the quest to reduce pain:

- Progesterone stimulates bone building cells (osteoblasts), and can affect nerve conduction.
- Estrogen alters the receptive properties of important nerves and inhibits resorption of bone. Estrogen and progesterone impact serotonin and other neurotransmitter levels.
- Vitamin B6 increases pain resistance.
- Calcium and magnesium are essential for electrolyte balance and bone building.
- Vitamin D influences absorption and retention of calcium (among many other things).
- Magnesium helps with migraines and PMS headaches.

Always talk with your healthcare practitioner to decide on the treatment approaches that are best suited for you.

Medications and Pain

In some medical conditions, medication is essential for the management of pain. The body is in a state of stress when pain is untreated, and untreated pain leads frequently to depression and listlessness which perpetuates the state of stress. The use of pain medication is a huge topic and beyond the scope of this book, so talk to your practitioner about a treatment protocol that meets your pain needs as you also begin to add in other treatments that help with any longer term underlying problems.

Stress and Pain

The neurotransmitters norepinephrine (noradrenaline) and epinephrine (adrenaline), are mediators of the stress response. Their role is to put the brain/body on alert, to be ready to flee or fight or freeze. When there is persistent pain there is potential to cause continual production of adrenaline, and then the stage is set for a potential long term stress response that can eventually lead to adrenal dysfunction. Stress can elevate the level of the neurotransmitter glutamate, and yet glutamate is known to increase activity in the pain neurons, thus increasing sensitivity to painful stimuli still further. Evaluating your neurotransmitter levels will give your healthcare practitioner valuable information on where to begin targeted treatment approaches designed specifically for you.

Additional solutions for resetting the systems and handling pain.

Chiropractic

Chiropractic is a health care profession that focuses on disorders of the musculoskeletal system and the nervous system, and the effects of these disorders on general health. Chiropractic care is used most often to treat neuro-musculoskeletal complaints, including but not limited to: back pain, neck pain, pain in the joints of the arms or legs, and headaches. Practitioners of Chiropractic, often referred to as chiropractors or chiropractic physicians, practice a drug-free, hands-on approach to health care that includes patient examination, diagnosis and treatment. Chiropractors have broad diagnostic skills and are also trained to recommend therapeutic and rehabilitative exercises, as well as to provide nutritional, dietary and lifestyle counseling. A chiropractor is not a licensed physician and has not completed residency training in a hospital.

The most common therapeutic procedure performed by practitioners of chiropractic is known as "spinal manipulation," also called "chiro-

-practic is known as "spinal manipulation," also called "chiropractic adjustment." The purpose of manipulation is to restore joint mobility by manually applying a controlled force into joints that have become restricted in their movement as a result of a tissue injury. Tissue injury can be caused by a single traumatic event, such as improper lifting of a heavy object, or through repetitive stresses, such as sitting in an awkward position with poor spinal posture for an extended period of time. In either case, injured tissues undergo physical and chemical changes that can cause inflammation, pain, and reduced function. Adjustment of the affected joint and tissues restores mobility, thereby alleviating pain and muscle tightness, and allowing tissues to heal. Chiropractic adjustment rarely causes discomfort. However, sometimes there may be mild soreness or aching following treatment (as with some forms of exercise) that usually goes away within twelve to forty-eight hours.

In many cases, such as lower back pain, chiropractic care may be the primary method of treatment. When other medical conditions exist, chiropractic care may complement or support medical treatment by relieving the musculoskeletal aspects associated with the condition. Chiropractors may assess patients through clinical examination, laboratory testing, diagnostic imaging such as ultrasound, and other tools to determine when chiropractic treatment is the right fit. Chiropractors will readily refer you to the appropriate health care practitioner when chiropractic care is not suitable at that time, or your particular health condition needs co-management in partnership with other healthcare practitioners.

Osteopathy

Osteopathic physicians understand how all the body's systems are interconnected and how each one affects the others. They receive special training in the musculoskeletal system so that they better understand how that system influences the condition of all other body systems. In addition, Doctors of Osteopathy (DO's) are trained to identify and correct structural problems, which can assist your body's natural tendency toward health and self-healing. Osteopathy also offers the added benefit of hands-on diagnosis and treatment through a system of therapy known as osteopathic manipulative treatment (OMT). DOs are complete physicians, fully trained and licensed to prescribe medicine and to perform surgery. With OMT, osteopathic physicians use their hands to diagnose illness and injury and encourage the body to heal itself. By combining all other appropriate medical options with OMT, DOs offer their patients very comprehensive care. The primary differences between a DO and a chiropractor are their levels of training and the scope of their practice.

Acupuncture

The classical Chinese explanation of acupuncture is that channels of energy run in regular patterns through the body and over its surface. These energy channels, called meridians, are like rivers flowing through the body carrying energy to irrigate and nourish the tissues. An obstruction in the movement of these energy rivers is like a dam that backs up a river. The energy can be blocked, deficient, excessive, or unbalanced. This throws Yin (the feminine aspect of life) and Yang (the masculine counterpart) out of balance, which in turn causes illness. Acupuncture frees up the flow of energy with the intention of encouraging the body to promote natural healing and to improve functioning. Tiny little needles are inserted into the skin at very precise acupuncture points on the meridians to unblock energy. Acupuncture can therefore restore balance and energy flow, thereby encouraging healing.

Needling the acupuncture points also stimulates the nervous system to release a soup of chemicals in the muscles, spinal cord and brain. As noted earlier in the chapter, these chemicals will either change the experience of pain, or they can trigger the release of other chemicals and hormones which influence the body's own internal regulating system. The improved energy and biochemical balance produced by acupuncture results in stimulating the body's natural healing abilities, and in promoting physical and emotional well-being.

Ayurveda

Ayurvedic medicine – also known as Ayurveda – is one of the world's oldest holistic (whole-body) healing systems. It developed thousands of years ago in India and is based on the belief that health and wellness depend on a delicate balance between the mind, body, and spirit. The primary focus of Ayurvedic medicine is to promote good health, rather than fight disease, however, treatments may be recommended for specific health problems.

Healing Touch

Healing Touch is a relaxing, nurturing energy therapy that uses gentle touch to assist in balancing physical, mental, emotional, and spiritual well-being. Healing Touch works with the human energy field to support the natural ability to heal, is safe for all ages, and works in harmony with naturopathic or allopathic medical care. There are a variety of healing touch modalities including: Healing Touch, Reiki, Qigong, and therapeutic touch; all are intended to affect energy fields within and around the body.

Energy Medicine – Energy in the Body

The entire body is a mass of tiny electrical currents that result from the chemical reactions that occur as part of the normal bodily functions. As you might remember from physics class, everything is made up of atoms, and an atom is made of a nucleus surrounded by an electron shell. In the nucleus are protons which are positively charged and neutrons which have no charge, hence their names. Each electron in the electron shell has a negative charge and they balance the positive charges in the nucleus. Atoms, and the molecules into which they combine, are normally in balance or equilibrium. The introduction of an extra electron starts an exchange process from atom to atom as electrons are nudged along the row. Imagine a row of basketball players sitting on a bench. If another player is added to one end of the already full bench everyone has to nudge the next player to move up. This flow of nudges is like the flow that goes from atom to atom when an extra electron is added, and the flow is what creates a current. The player at the other end gets excited because there is a risk of falling off.

Because the body is a huge masses of atoms, we can generate electricity. Electricity is a key to survival. Electrical signals are fast. They allow for a nearly instantaneous response to control messages. If the body relied entirely on, say, the slower movement of chemicals to tell the heart to speed up when something is chasing us, we would not be here today as a species. Most biochemical reactions, from digestion to brain activities, involve constant rearrangement of charged particles. All this moving around and reorganizing generates the exchange of positive and negative charges which creates a current of electricity. Everything we do is controlled and enabled by electrical signals running through the body.

Electricity in Wound Healing

Originally the role of electricity in wound healing did not receive much attention, even after a German physiologist called Emil Du Bois-Reymond cut his arm and measured the electrical field across the wound in the mid-1800s. Time passed, some more researchers periodically looked into the role of energy in healing, but it wasn't until recently that scientists have found how the body harnesses the power of electricity to heal cuts and grazes – in effect, scientists worked out how to manipulate energy to speed up the rate at which a wound heals. Researchers showed that by controlling the weak electrical fields that arise naturally at wound sites, they could direct cells to either close or open up a wound at the flick of a switch. By making the cells move faster, they were able to speed up wound healing by as much as fifty percent.

Russian scientists had been looking at electricity and energy in the body. Driven by the pressure of the space race, researchers were seeking a way to keep cosmonauts healthy while they were on long missions in space. Surgery requires complex machinery for which there was no room in a space craft; medications are so specific that how could they pick the right ones to take? Instead of traditional solutions, Russian scientists decided they needed a completely different mechanism capable of responding to both acute and chronic medical conditions. They eventually developed an energetic biofeedback device.

Several brands of these devices now exist and they all have very similar principles being small, hand held devices with transdermal (across skin) electro-stimulators. The device delivers non-invasive, computer modulated therapeutic electro-stimulation via the skin and involves high amplitude, short duration waveforms which are hardly felt at all. The device stimulates the small c-fibers to trigger the release of chemicals which leads to pain relief and healing. The device impulse is carried via "inbound" nerve fibers to regulatory centers in the brain which in turn responds via "outbound" nerve fibers to the wound location. The nerve responses going backwards and forwards between the damaged area and the brain are monitored constantly and, via a tiny computer inside, the electrical charges adjust constantly. As this process continues, the brain either amplifies or dampens the body's signals that cause pain, ultimately leading to homeostasis (balance) and healing.

As we know, points on the skin correspond to different meridians and organs in the body – these are the meridians that acupuncture uses.

The device can be used along meridian points to help determine the specific locations needing energetic intervention and then can provide a healing energy pattern to these areas. In acute situations the signal from the device focuses the brain on acute inflamed areas for more rapid healing and pain relief. For internal chronic pain, this technology can also stimulate the healing response to the right area using meridian lines.

This capacity for biofeedback is unique, it is as if the device is engaging in energetic conversation with the body and thus, it can teach the body to heal itself. The device sends out a series of signals through the skin and measures the response. Each signal is only sent out when a change, in response to the previous signal, is recorded in the electrical properties of the skin. The c-fibers, which comprise eighty five percent of all nerves in the body, react most readily to the electro-stimulation and are responsible for the production of neuropeptides and other regulatory peptides. By stimulation of the c-fibers, the device increases the levels of peptides available for the body to use where necessary. It is these neuropeptides that in turn re-establish the body's natural physiological state and so are responsible for the healing process. Because these peptides last up to several hours, the healing process will continue long after the treatment is over. The large quantity of neuropeptides and c-fibers in the CNS can also result in the treatment on one area aiding with other chemical imbalances, correcting sleeplessness, appetite and behavioral problems. A list of energetic biofeedback device manufacturers can be found in Appendix G.

Stepping into Health

So how can you stop the cycles of chronic pain? How do you reset the switches on your permanently "on" inflammatory immune response? The first step is to accept that, with the exception of traumatic injury situations, it probably took you a number of years to reach a state of chronic pain, and so it is unlikely that it will take a matter of minutes or some pills, to reset the process. However, there are plenty of things that you can do, individually and, more importantly collectively, with your healthcare practitioner to begin to undo patterns and forge new ones.

- Get adequate sleep
- Increase your intake of antioxidants
- Remove inflammatory foods

- Speed the healing process
- Undertake Energetic readjustments
- Make lifestyle changes
- Get healthy exercise
- Build your connection to your spirit and bring your mind to a state of peace

This chapter is designed to explain some of the basics of biochemistry and how pain and inflammation occurs. With this information you are now in a more informed place to discuss long term treatment approaches with your healthcare practitioner. For most long term chronic pain patients, there is no magic pill, however, there are lots of small changes that you can make that will help reduce inflammation and start the path back to health. Integrative Medicine practitioners consider that disease is due to lack of balance within the body systems. Establishing proper balance by employing the above nutrients, therapies, and lifestyle modifications may thus offer a safe and effective alternative to conventional treatment and bring new hope to patients suffering from long term chronic dis-ease.

Chapter Four Summary – Pain

- The role of pain and inflammation
- The natural process of healing after damage
- The nervous, endocrine and immune systems
- Free radical damage
- Common disease states that result in chronic pain: Crohn's, ulcerative colitis, joint pain, back pain, arthritis.
- Headaches and migraines
- The role of exercise in pain management
- Inflammatory and Anti-Inflammatory foods
- Alternative solutions: chiropractic, osteopathy, acupuncture, ayurveda, healing touch
- Energy Medicine in the body
- Stepping into health

CHAPTER FIVE

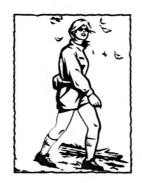

EXERCISE

Hopefully after reading this chapter you will see the word exercise and smile more often than groan. I love exercise, but even as I am sitting here starting to write this chapter I groaned at the thought of heading to the pool to swim. My body hurts – I did way, way too much last weekend building a section of deck, and my body has ached all week in consequence. I shamelessly used the excuse that my left hip and lower back are too inflamed to avoid exercise all this week. And I feel like a slug. What my body and mind need most is, in fact, exercise. Okay – I am off to the pool. I will be right back.

It worked, as it does, just about every time. An hour of exercise using my muscles and lungs makes a world of difference to how my body feels. In fact, the pain in my hip has gone. How can that be? Well, endorphins are a big part of the answer. When we move around vigorously, exercising multiple muscles for a period of time, this causes a small amount of stress. Good, healthy stress. As the muscles are used, tiny tears in the muscle will appear. Endorphins are produced in response to the stress and act as analgesics, which means they diminish the perception of pain. The neuron receptors that endorphins bind to are the same ones that bind some pain medicines. However, unlike with morphine, the activation of these receptors by the body's endorphins does not usually lead to addiction or dependence. That is a good thing.

So, think back to what you read in the previous Chapter on Pain. When there is damage to the body in any way, the immune system kicks into overdrive releasing inflammatory cytokines to remove the threat/broken parts and repair the damage. Blood flow will increase across all the tissues in the body, and gradually capillary networks will expand. The more blood networks there are in the body, the quicker the delivery of oxygen is to the body and the faster the removal of waste products out. The body is automatically removing the broken bits and rebuilding new parts, at a micro level.

Exercise improves the pumping action of the heart, and regular exercise will actually help expand the system of veins and arteries and capillaries in the body, allowing for increased blood flow. The improved blood flow means that more toxins and waste are cleaned out from various parts of the body through sweating and exhaling. Because thirst rises with exercise, increased intake of water to quench that thirst will also help with removing toxins from the body. Exercise can be a very effective way to create the right amount of stress to promote healing.

As you know, the body is always healing itself: cells die in programmed time, the body has mechanisms to clean out what is broken/damaging/toxic, and then rebuild and regrow. As we get older the repair work isn't as efficient as it used to be so it is increasingly important to exercise to help ensure the "destroy and repair" process occurs consistently. Yes, I worked too hard on the deck and set up inflammation in a couple, well, several of my muscles and joints, but after a few day's rest, it would have been better for me to start exercising again to help the healing process.

As mentioned above, the biggest impact of exercise is on the health of the heart. The heart is like the engine of a car. Without the engine working, the car isn't going anywhere. If the engine isn't lubricated well, the car won't work well, and will likely seize up. The heart is an amazing organ, we need it to beat at least sixty times a minute, for every minute of an hour, of a day, of a week, month, year, of our lives. Unlike leg muscles, which get a rest when we lie down and go to sleep, we need our hearts to keep on going and going and going. When stressed through exercise, the heart grows stronger and larger. If not stressed as a result of an inactive lifestyle, the heart will get smaller and smaller, just like other muscles. A strong heart has the ability to circulate blood throughout the entire body with ease. The stronger the pumping capacity the greater the flow of blood throughout all the organs, limbs, and extremities such as fingers and toes. With proper exercise the heart becomes more massive and powerful, and more efficient. A well-conditioned heart beats more slowly at rest and during work, and builds a greater pumping capacity. When the heart relaxes, the cambers of the heart fill with blood, then, when the heart muscles contract it pumps hard to force the blood out into the arteries. This is the best exercise the heart can get. A heart made strong by exercise will pump blood more efficiently and with less strain.

Exercise provides the heart with a secondary support system. Every muscle in the body also helps to pump blood, and muscles pump blood back to the heart. When a muscle elsewhere in the body muscle relaxes, that muscle will be filled with blood. When the muscle then contacts, it squeezes blood back towards the heart. A person carrying an extra ten pounds of muscle is not straining their heart with the extra poundage, they are actually working in support of the heart. If someone carries an extra ten pounds of fat, then the heart will be taxed, the fat does nothing to help with the flow of blood and it also carries millions of parasitic capillaries that need to be serviced with blood. A sedentary lifestyle means that blood vessels will very likely close up, shrink, and maybe disappear. The great news is that getting back to exercise reserves this trend, and relatively quickly.

The lower the resting heart rate, the lower the risk of coronary heart disease. A resting heart rate will be about fifteen to twenty beats per minute lower than when walking around. During rest, the parasympathetic branch of the autonomic nervous system keeps the rate low. As soon as the body moves, the sympathetic branch kicks in, releasing epinephrine (adrenaline) which creates an electrical charge to the heart muscle (like the ignition on a car). The electrical charge will increase the heart rate, breathing rate, and blood pressure. It is essential that the heart is regularly sparked into working harder so that it stays strong and capable of beating.

Here is a tough statistic: more women die of heart disease each year than from all of the cancers combined. A sedentary lifestyle will increase the rate of death through heart disease by five times. Although we hear about heart failure as a cause of death, it is not actually the heart that fails to work, it is the coronary arteries that stop working. Coronary arteries are the mechanism that supplies blood to the actual heart muscle. Maintaining the muscles of the heart is very important, it is like maintaining the engine of a car. As mentioned before, if the engine seizes up – you can't go anywhere. If a heart seizes up due to poor muscle tone and/or blocked arteries then, well, it is curtains time. Taking care of the heart is essential for survival.

How does a heart become damaged?

White blood cells circulate through all arteries all the time, on guard to absorb cholesterol and clean up the blood stream. When someone eats a diet consistently high in cholesterol, the extra cholesterol builds up to form plaque on the artery wall. The coronary (heart) arteries are the mechanism for feeding blood to the heart muscle itself – the muscle that will drive the pump action of all four chambers of the heart. A buildup of plaque causes the coronary arteries to gradually harden and eventually small cracks appear. Even a tiny crack in the artery wall signals the need to "stop the bleeding" and so the immune system, charging to the rescue, makes a clot form around the crack. If it is a big enough clot, the artery will be blocked and so now blood cannot flow to that part of the heart. Without blood flow, the heart muscle stops and there is a heart attack. If the cracks are small, the repair clots are small enough to allow blood to continue to flow through the artery, however, over time, repeated clots will gradually narrow the artery and make it harder and harder to keep blood circulating.

Toxins that are damaging to the body can enter the blood stream through a number of places – through cuts and abrasions, through sores and ulcers, or through holes in the gut. Blood returning to the heart will carry those toxins through the heart. The immune system will be working hard to neutralize and then excrete the toxins, but if there are a lot, then toxins can be lodged in the heart and then cause localized inflammation.

We know from Chapter Three on Nutrition that there are many things that can be done to reduce the level of cholesterol in the blood-stream – eating cruciferous vegetables, adding salads, avocado, cold water fish; reducing red meat, saturated fats, sugar, etc. Partnering tasty and healthy food choices with exercise that gradually builds strength and stamina is the way to rebuild heart health. Of course, the type of exercise chosen depends on the starting point and what goals someone wants to achieve. Always discuss your options for exercise with your practitioner to make sure you start at a sensible place for your current state of health.

The next page is a list of benefits of exercise. When you read the list it is an easy step to realize that humans are designed to move. Moving is as natural and as necessary as breathing. Return in your mind to the cave dwelling days. Hunting and gathering required moving. Deer did not turn up at the cave bearing a note that said "take out has arrived, delivered in under thirty minutes", they had to be tracked and chased. Bushes and trees containing food were spread out, animals were sneaky and hid, so our brains and bodies developed in symphony to solve the problem of getting food. Again, although thousands and thousands of years have passed, and we can order pizza and groceries to be delivered to our door so we never have to move to find food, our bodies still have the same biochemistry as our ancestors. We are wired to move, and our health and wellness depends on us moving frequently.

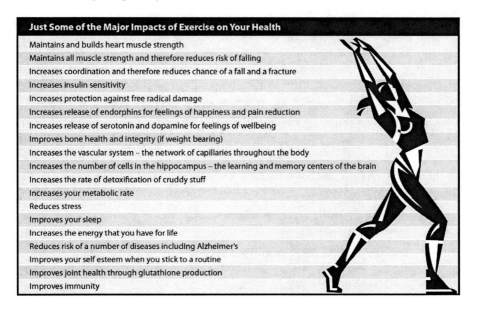

Just Some of the Major Impacts of Exercise on Your Health
Maintains and builds heart muscle strength
Maintains all muscle strength and therefore reduces risk of falling
Increases coordination and therefore reduces chance of a fall and a fracture
Increases insulin sensitivity
Increases protection against free radical damage
Increases release of endorphins for feelings of happiness and pain reduction
Increases release of serotonin and dopamine for feelings of wellbeing
Improves bone health and integrity (if weight bearing)
Increases the vascular system – the network of capillaries throughout the body
Increases the number of cells in the hippocampus – the learning and memory centers of the brain
Increases the rate of detoxification of cruddy stuff
Increases your metabolic rate
Reduces stress
Improves your sleep
Increases the energy that you have for life
Reduces risk of a number of diseases including Alzheimer's
Improves your self esteem when you stick to a routine
Improves joint health through glutathione production
Improves immunity

The Impact of Exercise on Mood

If I am feeling a little down for any reason, I know that exercise will help. Years ago I used to be easily irritated and angry and I found that going to the pool to swim made a huge difference to my mood. Even now, if something has come up that has me thrown off center, I know that swimming laps for thirty to forty-five minutes, or taking a long walk around the hills in my neighborhood will help settle my brain and allow me to relax and see what it is that I need to see. There is still no clear agreement on how exercise improves mood, studies are on-going, but enough research now has shown that exercise for thirty to forty-five minutes three times a week can be at least as effective for long and short term depression as antidepressants.

Detoxification and Free Radicals

Remember free radicals? A free radical is an atom or group of atoms with at least one unpaired electron. In the body, it is usually an oxygen molecule that has lost an electron and needs to stabilize itself by stealing an electron from a nearby molecule. That thieving process is called oxidation. Whatever the free radical touches first (and steals the electron from), is wrecked. If it is the cell wall, the cell dies. If it is the DNA, it causes a mutation – and that can easily lead to a range of diseases, including cancer.

Free radicals only last for a tiny fraction of a second, but during their fleeting existence, they cause some serious structural damage to your cells. Much like a tornado passing through Kansas, free radicals often leave a huge path of destruction in their wake. Once a molecule is oxidized by the free radical, it often starts a chain reaction of oxidation that continues until an antioxidant can stop it. That is why free radicals and antioxidants must go hand in hand. Regular physical exercise enhances the antioxidant defense system and protects against exercise induced free radical damage as well as other free radical damage. Glutathione – a major antioxidant, is produced during exercise.

Be wary though, intense exercise for an untrained body overwhelms defenses resulting in increased free radical damage. If someone is sedentary during the week but then engages in vigorous bouts of exercise during the weekend it may be doing more harm than good, including dumping a bunch of free radicals into the body.

Bone Health

High impact weight bearing exercise will build bone, so does strength training. Bone grows and replaces itself every two years. With aging, gradually more bone is lost than made, unless lifestyle involves an exercise routine that includes weight bearing activity. The goal is to build more bone than is lost naturally. Increased muscle strength and coordination will improve balance and, with aging, will help reduce the chances of falling and breaking a bone, which then takes a long time to repair. The longer someone is down after a fracture, the more muscle and bone wasting occurs. My older daughter fractured her right tibial plateau during a ski race and by the time she came off crutches, the muscles in her right leg were thirty percent smaller than her left leg. And that was age sixteen. At forty-six, or fifty-six or sixty-six, that proportionate wasting is much greater.

Exercise and Hormones

Exercise will help regulate cortisol production making it less likely that surging cortisol levels will contribute to constant feelings of anxiety and a growing waistline. Studies also suggest that exercise can help reduce estrogen levels and increase the binding globulin that binds up free estrogen. This is important because as we get older, both men and women will frequently have excess estrogen. Exercise also plays an important role in regulating insulin within the body. During exercise, glucose is used to power muscles. Because glucose levels drop, less insulin is required to be released from the pancreas. Be wary however if you have diabetes and are using insulin; it is absolutely critical that you discuss your insulin dose with your practitioner, because the amount and type of exercise you choose to do will impact the amount of insulin your body will need.

Sleep

Exercising vigorously right before bed or within about three hours of your bedtime can actually make it harder to fall asleep. This surprises many people; it is often thought that a good workout before bed helps you feel more tired. In actuality, vigorous exercise right before bed stimulates the heart, brain and muscles – the opposite of what is wanted at bedtime. It also raises body temperature right before bed, which is not ideal.

Morning exercise can relieve stress and improve mood. These effects can indirectly improve sleep, no doubt. To get a more direct sleep-promoting benefit from morning exercise, however, you can couple it with exposure to outdoor light. Being exposed to natural light in the morning, whether exercising or not, can improve sleep at night by reinforcing the body's sleep-wake cycle. We know that exercise releases endorphins which can act as sedatives. They are manufactured in the brain, spinal cord, and many other parts of the body and are released in response to brain chemicals called neurotransmitters.

When it comes to having a direct effect on getting a good night's sleep, it is vigorous exercise in the late afternoon or early evening that appears most beneficial. That is because it raises body temperature above normal a few hours before bed, allowing it to start falling just as bedtime rolls around. This decrease in body temperature appears to be a trigger that helps ease into sleep.

The type of vigorous workout we're talking about to help sleep is a cardiovascular workout. That means engaging in some activity in which the heart rate is raised and muscles are pumping continuously for at least twenty minutes. Although strength-training, stretching, yoga and other methods of exercise are beneficial, none match the sleep-enhancing benefits of cardiovascular exercise.

Brain Health

Exercise improves learning on three levels: it optimizes mindset by improving alertness, attention, and motivation; it prepares and encourages nerve cells to bind to one another, which is the cellular basis for learning new information; and it spurs the development of new nerve cells from stem cells in the hippocampus, an area of the brain related to memory and learning. How can this be? Exercise increases production of the neurotransmitter dopamine, which affects attention and learning; and norepinephrine, which influences attention, perception, motivation and arousal. fMRI studies have shown that exercise increases blood flow to the part of the hippocampus that is involved in memory formation. This impact of exercise lasts about three days and then it begins to fade, thus it is important to exercise regularly to maintain the benefits. Increased blood flow also allows more nutrients in and faster detoxification out. It is also very likely that exercise stimulates a chemical called Brain Derived Neurotrophic Factor (BDNF), which is responsible for developing healthy brain tissue.

So, if exercise is good for us, is doing no exercise bad for the brain? Yes, absolutely. Lack of regular exercise will undoubtedly impact the brain. The central message of this chapter is "get blood flow up, and increase circulation of blood flow through the body to deliver oxygen and food and to take away the waste products". If good flow of blood to the brain is not maintained, the blood vessels in the brain get smaller and bent out of shape, which may increase the risk of tiny strokes where blood cannot flow easily through the brain. Not good.

Type of Exercise

Both cardiovascular and resistive exercise are important. Cardiovascular exercise improves the pumping strength of the heart and resistive exercise builds up muscle strength. Repeated, long slow steady exercise is what is necessary to counter the impacts of inflammation. Higher intensity exercise will build strength and increase muscle power and maintain the nerve network throughout your body. Both are important, so the ideal routine combines both. Keeping legs strong is important – they are needed to support the body and help maintain balance and avoid falls that could result in a fractured hip. Thigh muscles replace themselves every four months, so long gaps of inactivity will result in muscle wasting quite quickly. Always warm up to allow the heart and circulatory system to prepare for exercise, and always warm down to keep blood circulating and not pooling at the ankles.

The purpose of exercise as discussed here is to improve and maintain body and brain functions for optimal health. Effort is the energy you expend, work is the physical action that effort produces. You can evaluate both by monitoring your pulse rate. There are four things that you can feel when sensing your pulse.

1. The first is the force of the pulse against your fingers. As you become fit, this force gets stronger.
2. The second is the volume, or expansion of the artery. As you become fit, the volume increases, and the artery feels thicker, yet soft and elastic.
3. The third is the regularity of the force and the rhythm. As you become fit, your pulse becomes stronger and more regular.
4. The fourth is frequency. As you become fit, the frequency of pulse beat reduces.

Strong muscles can squeeze a lot of blood out of the heart muscle fibers, weak muscles squeeze only a little. A weak heart has to work harder (beat faster) to circulate blood. The goal of exercise is to reduce the resting pulse/heart rate. The lower your resting heart rate, the lower the risk of coronary heart disease. Exercise strengthens the heart so that it performs more efficiently at lower rates by (i) improving the quality of the heart muscle and (ii) increasing the coordination of the fibers as they wring blood out of the heart each beat.

Fat Burning Zone

There are two sources of fuel for exercise: fat and glycogen. Glycogen is a form of carbohydrate stored in the muscles. Fat is packed in cells and stored all over the body. Both fat and glycogen are used to provide energy. When the heart is working at lower rates fat will be burned; at higher rates, more glycogen will be burned to meet the intense need. When exercising at a slower rate, fewer calories will be used per unit of time. Higher intensity exercise burns more calories and, even though a higher proportion comes from utilizing glycogen, the higher demand burns more fat. Higher intensity exercise does also increase metabolic rate for anything from a few minutes to a few hours after it is ended, so calories continue to burn at a faster rate.

Now, fat is not stored in the muscles where it is needed, fat is stored (as we all know) in places like the hips, thighs, stomach. Fat is moved from storage to the muscles by triglycerides. Triglycerides are then broken down into free fatty acids which can be used for energy, and also into glycerol, which can be converted to glucose for brain energy. Your practitioner may measure your triglyceride levels – high levels are associated with increased risk of heart disease. Regular exercise will "burn up" those triglycerides and help your heart.

Conclusion

If you have been sedentary for a long time, ask your practitioner for recommendations on exercise or for a referral to someone who can help. You may need to use the resources around the home to get exercise; others may join a gym; some people can afford a private coach to help start a program. When I travel in winter, I will sometimes get my daily dose of aerobic weight bearing exercise by walking up and down the twenty flights of stairs in the hotel. It can be grubby and boring, but I put a story on my Ipod and off I go for thirty minutes or more. If you have been injured or have long term joint pain, then physical therapy can be the starting point to restoring function and fitness.

Exercise doesn't have to be a workout at the gym or a thirty mile bike ride, keeping active in your yard, walking with friends in the park, going dancing, are all wonderful ways to keep moving. I love to build things, I love power tools, and a Saturday will often find me outside building something for several hours on end. After a good breakfast around 8 a.m. I can sometimes be on the go until 2 p.m. when my body finally reminds me that "lunch would be good here." Those active days, carrying lumber, getting up and down off ladders, bending and stooping, holding equipment, pressing hard with all muscles, increases my metabolic rate, the movement triggers energy burning and it takes longer for me to feel hungry. In contrast, I can have the same size breakfast on a weekday, get to work, sit like a stone at my desk focused on my computer, and be hungry after three hours.

There are beautiful stories on any number of TV channels these days of wonderful women who decided that even though the path back to wellness was a tough one, they just had to start. Many people who have not been exercising will start with walking. It is free, it is always there, it can start gently and gradually build up to a greater level of intensity. The key thing is to start, even if it hurts in the beginning.

Which exercise plan is the best? There is no absolute answer to this. It is all about scale. If you are doing nothing – anything is better than nothing. If you are doing some exercise, then getting more vigorous exercise is better. If you are already active – then look to add in a mix of strength training and endurance exercise. Fitness is a lifestyle that has amazing benefits for your heart, your brain, your mood, your sleep and for everyone around you.

Chapter Five Summary – Exercise

- Impact of exercise on the heart
- Importance of heart health
- Impact of exercise on mood
- Impact of exercise on detoxification
- Bone, hormones, sleep and brain health
- Exercise options
- Role of exercise in fat burning processes

CHAPTER SIX

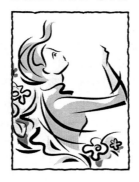

TOXICITY

At every turn these days it seems we hear about a new detox diet that claims you can clean your body and lose ten pounds in five days or even twenty pounds in a month. So enticing, so interesting, so hopeful. In addition there are so many blenders and juicers and fasts, it is hard to know which is the best way to go. While detoxification can certainly have the side effect of weight loss, for centuries, many holistic practitioners have understood that the greater value of detoxification is overall physical and emotional vitality.

Our bodies are energy-making and energy-burning organisms and, just like a car engine, anytime we make and burn energy, or perform some function, waste is created. The body has evolved efficient ways to eliminate that waste: nutrients come in and are processed; toxic wastes are produced and then eliminated. We are detoxing all the time. Even in the most pristine of environments, with the most perfect balance of diet, exercise, water and sleep, the body is always detoxing. The purpose of detoxification is to remove from the body that which can cause harm: products of metabolism, excess hormones, vitamins, inflammatory molecules, heavy metals, and other compounds.

Given that detoxification is a natural bodily function, why now is there so much in the media about detoxification and "doing a detox diet"? The answer to that question lies, as it does in most chapters in this book, in how humans have moved away from the "natural state" as human mammals, into a significantly more toxin and stress laden environment.

Toxins are poisonous compounds produced by living organisms. Sometimes the term "biotoxin" is used to emphasize the biological origin of these compounds. Man-made chemical compounds with toxic potential are more properly called toxicants. Toxins and toxicants can exert their detrimental effects on health in a number of ways. Some broadly act as mutagens or carcinogens causing DNA damage (mutations), which can lead to diseases including cancer; others can disrupt specific metabolic pathways which can lead to the dysfunction of particular biological systems such as the nervous system, liver, or kidneys.

The diet is a major source of toxin exposure. Toxins can find their way into food through several routes, notably contamination by microorganisms, man-made toxicants including pesticides, residues from food processing, prescription drugs, and industrial wastes. Some of the toxic heavy metals (such as lead, mercury, cadmium, chromium), while not "man-made," have been released and/or redistributed into the environment at potentially dangerous levels by humans, and can find their way into the diet as well. Microbial toxins, secreted by bacteria and fungi, can be ingested along with contaminated or improperly prepared food.

Even the method of food preparation has the potential for converting naturally-occurring food constituents into toxins. For instance, high temperatures can convert nitrogen-containing compounds in meats and cereal products into the powerful mutagens benzopyrene and acrylamide, respectively. Smoked fish and cheeses contain precursors to toxins called N-nitroso compounds (NOCs), which can then affect DNA when metabolized by bacteria in the colon. Outside of the diet, breathing in volatile organic compounds (VOCs) is a common risk which has been associated with several adverse health effects, including kidney damage, immunological problems, hormonal imbalances, blood disorders, and increased rates of asthma and bronchitis.

Unfortunately, one of the greatest sources of non-dietary toxicant exposure is the air in the home. Building materials (such as floor and wall coverings, particle board, adhesives, and paints) can "off-gas," releasing several toxicants that can be detected in humans. Newly built or remodeled buildings can have substantial amounts of chemical "off-gassing", leading to what has been called "sick building syndrome." Carpet is an especially big offender, potentially releasing several neurotoxins. Carpets also trap environmental toxins, and infants and toddlers and short people are particularly at risk because they spend so much time close to carpet.

Understanding this internal body cleaning process involves exploring some more biochemistry. Every single one of the billions of cells in the body has a waterproof sac around it called a membrane. Cell membranes are most frequently composed of a fatty substance which does not easily allow a water-based molecule to pass through it (remember that oil and water do not mix). Any toxins that are dissolved in water are therefore unable to enter the cell and this makes a great protective mechanism. However, many of the toxic chemicals that enter the body are fat-soluble, which means they dissolve in fatty or oily solutions. Toxins that are dissolved in fat-based molecules can easily pass through the cell membrane and into the cell, rather like entering a nightclub holding the hand of someone in the "In-crowd" – the door magically opens. However, here's the kicker, the toxin, wrapped in a fatty substance, cannot easily pass back out through the cell membrane, (once inside the nightclub it is hard to get out). This easy transport into the cell makes it difficult for the body to excrete the toxins.

Fat-soluble toxins/chemicals have a high affinity for fat tissues and cell membranes, which are composed of fatty acids and proteins. In these fatty tissues (and we all know where they are), toxins may be stored for years, and then can be released during times of exercise, stress or fasting. If toxins are released in large quantities, several symptoms, such as headaches, poor memory, stomach pain, nausea, fatigue, dizziness and palpitations, can occur. Toxins in cells can interfere with DNA in quite dangerous ways through causing mutations to the gene code.

This is clearly not good for the body's survival chances and, in response, the body developed mechanisms to remove toxins. Enzymes are the key to the removal process. Remember that enzymes are agents of change (catalysts) – they will cause a change in their target molecules. In the detoxification process, enzymes are responsible for converting the fat soluble toxin into a water-based toxin, ready for it to be ejected from the cell and then excreted through urine or bile. The conversion process happens in two phases followed by an elimination phase.

Phase One Detoxification – Transformation

Under most circumstances, Phase One enzymes begin the detoxification process by chemically transforming fat soluble compounds into water soluble compounds in preparation for Phase Two detoxification. The bulk of the Phase One processes are performed by a family of enzymes called the cytochrome P450s (CYPs). CYP enzymes have the potential to recognize and modify countless different toxins. CYPs are amongst the most well studied and best characterized detoxification proteins due to their role in the metabolism of both prescription drugs and internally produced biochemical toxins (biotoxins). Several other enzymes contribute to the Phase One process as well, notably: the flavin monooxygenases (FMOs; responsible for the detoxification of nicotine from cigarette smoke); alcohol and aldehyde dehydrogenases (which metabolize drinking alcohol), and monoamine oxidases (MAO's; which break down serotonin, dopamine, and epinephrine in neurons and are targets of several older antidepressant drugs).

Phase Two Detoxification – Enzymatic Conjugation

Following Phase One transformation, the original fat-soluble toxin has been converted into a more water-soluble form. However, it is still not quite ready for immediate elimination from the cell for a couple of reasons: 1) Phase One reactions are not sufficient to make the toxin water-soluble enough to complete the entire excretion pathway; and 2) in many cases, products from the Phase One reactions are often even more toxic than they were originally. If these reactive molecules are not further metabolized by Phase Two, they may cause damage to proteins, RNA and DNA within the cell. Phase Two enzymes therefore complete the modification of the molecules so they can both leave the cell and be no longer "dangerous".

Phase Two is called the conjugation pathway, whereby the liver cells add another substance (eg. cysteine, glycine or a sulfur molecule) to a toxic substance to make it less harmful. The conjugation molecules are acted upon by specific enzymes to catalyze the reaction step. This makes the toxic substance completely water-soluble so it can be excreted from the cell and then from the body via watery fluids such as bile or urine. Through conjugation, the liver is able to turn drugs, hormones and various toxins into excretable substances. For efficient Phase Two detoxification, the liver cells require sulfur-containing amino acids such as taurine and cysteine. The micro-nutrients glycine, glutamine, choline and inositol are also required for efficient Phase Two detoxification. The diagram below shows the three main Phase Two enzyme groups and their main functions.

Enzyme Group	Function
UDP-glucuronlytransferases	Attach glucoronic acid to toxins to make them less reactive and more water soluble. Most are located in the liver.
Glutathione S-transferases	Major role in metabolism of bio-toxins produced by natural processes of metabolism. Present throughout the body.
Sulfortransferases	Attach a sulfur molecule to toxins - notably drugs and atmospheric toxicants.

Balancing the Phases of Detoxification

The rate at which Phase One occurs must be balanced by the rate at which Phase Two finishes its processing. People with a very active Phase One detoxification system but who have slow or inactive Phase Two enzymes are termed pathological detoxifiers. These people suffer unusually severe toxic reactions to environmental poisons. If you need to undergo detoxification treatment, your practitioner may do a liver detoxification test to pinpoint exactly how efficiently your liver is carrying out the detoxification process and find out if you are a pathological detoxifier.

An imbalance between Phase One and Phase Two can also occur when a person is exposed to large amounts of toxins or exposed to toxins for a long period of time. In these situations, the critical nutrients needed for Phase Two detoxification are usually depleted, which allows the highly toxic activated substances to build up.

Phase Three Detoxification – Transport

Phase Three transporters are present in many tissues, including the liver, intestines, kidneys, and brain, where they can provide a barrier against toxin entry, and a mechanism for actively moving toxins out of cells. Phase Three transporters actively pump toxins through the cell membrane and out of the cell, (think of them as bouncers in the nightclub escorting a poorly behaving patron out onto the street). In the liver, Phase Three transporters move glutathione, sulfate, and glucuronide conjugates out of cells into the bile for elimination. In the kidney and intestine, Phase Three transporters can remove xenobiotics from the blood for excretion from the body in urine and stool.

Proper functioning of the liver's detoxification systems is especially important for the prevention of cancer. A high proportion of all cancers are thought to be due to the effects of environmental carcinogens, such as those in cigarette smoke, food, water, and air, combined with deficiencies of the nutrients the body needs for proper functioning of the detoxification and immune systems. The level of exposure to environmental carcinogens varies widely, as does the efficiency of the detoxification enzymes, particularly Phase Two. High levels of exposure to carcinogens coupled with slow detoxification enzymes significantly increases susceptibility to cancer.

When optimum nutrition is provided, the liver operates efficiently. Many (and perhaps most) people do not eat the right kinds of foods to provide the liver with everything it needs for the elimination of the extra toxins that the body is exposed to daily. If nutrition is compromised through poor dietary and lifestyle habits, this will hinder detoxification processes, and other organs will suffer as the body retains these toxins. When working properly, the liver clears ninety nine percent of the bacteria and other toxins during the first pass. However, when the liver is damaged, such as in alcoholics or those people with a genetic variant that leads to a damaged liver, the time it takes for toxins to clear increases by a factor of over ten.

As mentioned, the liver's Phase Two detoxification process involves the synthesis and secretion of a fluid substance called bile. Each day the liver manufactures approximately one quart of bile, which serves as a carrier in which many toxic substances are dumped into the intestines. Bile functions a bit like a detergent that picks up dirt, grease and oil. In the intestines, the bile and its toxic load are absorbed by fiber and excreted. However, a diet low in fiber results in poor binding and then reabsorption of the toxins. This problem is made worse when bacteria in the intestine modify these toxins to more damaging forms.

Several other mechanisms work in concert with the Phase One, Two, and Three systems to improve their efficiency or extend their functionality. While not officially part of xenobiotic metabolism, they are still important for reducing or modifying toxin exposure. The next diagram shows the flow of the detoxification process.

Other key elements of the detoxification process:

- Bile secretion is a critical digestive process for the absorption of dietary fats and fat-soluble nutrients, but it also functions as the major mechanism for moving toxins from Phase Two out of the liver and into the intestines where they can be eliminated.

- Antioxidation is a necessary protective measure against the harsh Phase One oxidation reactions, which frequently produce free-radical byproducts. Antioxidant enzymes are important for minimizing this free-radical damage. Antioxidants can be added to a detox diet to help reduce free-radical damage.

- Glutathione. Heavy metal toxicity can lead to oxidative damage by increasing free radicals and depleting antioxidant reserves. Glutathione is an important antioxidant, but mercury, arsenic, and lead, for example, effectively inactivate the glutathione molecule. Heavy metals will be discussed in more detail later in this chapter.

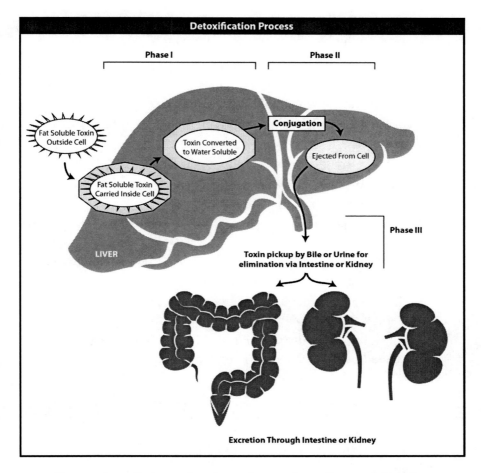

Detoxification Process

Phase I

Phase II

Fat Soluble Toxin Outside Cell

Fat Soluble Toxin Carried Inside Cell

Toxin Converted to Water Soluble

Conjugation

Ejected From Cell

Phase III

LIVER

Toxin pickup by Bile or Urine for elimination via Intestine or Kidney

Excretion Through Intestine or Kidney

- Prevention of absorption through trapping of potential toxins (such as sticking to another molecule in the gut, like activated charcoal or kaolin clay) is an effective means of moderating exposure; this mechanism has the requirement of some dietary adsorbent to be taken while the toxin is in transit in the GI tract. Uptake of potential toxins and their detoxification by beneficial bacteria in the colon could have a similar effect.

It is important to remember that the detoxification process has three distinct stages to it and that each stage can be impacted in different ways by the different actions we take. As mentioned above, if Phase One detoxification happens faster than Phase Two can handle, there will be a build-up of the converted toxic elements that can do more harm than the toxins them selves. Working with a practitioner on detoxification helps ensure that the detoxification method chosen does no harm.

The balance between the first two phases is influenced by many factors including, but not limited to the following:

- Diet. A diet low in fiber, high in processed foods and non-organic produce, will both increase the number of toxins in the body and reduce the rate at which toxins are released from the body.
- Smoking and alcohol consumption both increase Phase One detoxification.
- Age. As we age, the body's ability to detox declines.
- Genetics. We may have genetic defects that reduce the body's ability to detox normally.
- Disease. Some diseases can increase the uptake of toxins into the body.
- Drugs. Intake of both prescription and street drugs increase the rate of Phase One detoxification.
- Environment. Chemical and heavy metal toxic substances in air, soil, and water, all contribute to high levels of toxicity.
- Prolonged Stress. Negative emotional stress increases the number of free radicals which cause oxidative damage and increase biotoxin levels.

Phase One and Phase Two Detoxification Process	
Substances That Activate Phase One Detoxification	**Drugs:** alcohol; nicotine in cigarette smoke; Phenobarbital; sulfonamides; steroids
	Foods: cabbage, broccoli, and Brussel sprouts; charcoal-broiled meats; high-protein diet; oranges and tangerines (but not grapefruits)
	Nutrients: niacin; vitamin B1; vitamin C
	Herbs: caraway and dill seeds
	Environmental toxins: carbon tetrachloride; exhaust fumes; paint fumes; dioxin; pesticides
	Grapefruit juice, which contains naringenin, does however, slow down Phase One enzyme activity. It decreases the rate of elimination of drugs from the blood and has been found to substantially alter their clinical activity and toxicity. Eight ounces of grapefruit juice contains enough of the flavonoid naringenin to decrease cytochrome P450 activity by a remarkable 30%.
Substances That Activate Phase Two Detoxification	Compounds from citrus fruit and the Brassica or cruciferous group of vegetables (e.g., cabbage, Brussels sprouts, broccoli, etc.)
	Dietary supplements such as alpha-lipoic acid
	Green Tea
	Calcium D-glucarate
	Turmeric

Avoiding Toxin/Toxicant Exposure

While it is not possible to completely eliminate toxin/toxicant exposure from all sources, there are ways to minimize it:

- Limit the introduction of VOCs in the home by using VOC-free cleaning products, low-VOC paints, and choosing throw rugs instead of new carpeting.

- Check to make sure that Radon levels in the home are below the recommended level set by the EPA. (http://www.epa.gov/radon/pubs/citguide.html).

- Store food in bisphenolA (BPA)-free or phthalate-free containers and avoid reheating foods in plastic containers.

- Look for organic produce, which is grown without pesticides, and will contain less residue than conventionally-produced fruits and vegetables (although be aware that organic produce isn't necessarily "pesticide free").

- Washing fruits or vegetables can decrease some pesticide residue, although it is not effective against all pesticide types. Peeling skins off of produce may help to further lower pesticide levels.

- Limit intake of processed foods. Even foods that are free of synthetic preservatives may contain detectable amounts of toxic compounds that were introduced (by chemical transformation) during processing. For example, numerous toxins are produced by the high temperatures used to manufacture some processed food ingredients.

- Although the risk of acute toxicity from undercooking meat (food poisoning) is likely a greater risk than toxin exposure from overcooking it, there are ways to reduce toxin production during meat preparation: avoid direct exposure of meat to open flame or hot metal surfaces; cook meat at or below 250F via stewing, braising, crockpot cooking (slow food preparation methods that utilize liquid); turn meat often during cooking, avoid prolonged cooking time at high temperatures, and refrain from consuming charred portions. If you use a grill for cooking – turn food regularly to reduce charring and clean the grill frequently.

Oxidative Stress

You will recall that free radicals, also known as oxidants, are naturally formed but non-the-less harmful by-product's of natural cell metabolism that occurs in the human body on a continuous basis (e.g. from breathing, exercise, digestion). The normal molecules in the body contain electrons in pairs and this pairing of electrons is what makes the molecule stable. When a molecule loses one of its electrons, it becomes unstable, thereby a free radical is created. These are highly unstable molecules and, in an attempt to regain stability, they devour electrons from surrounding molecules. This creates more damaged molecules and, in a cascading effect, this leads to further more damaged cells, which causes degeneration of those cells. The destruction of healthy tissue that occurs as a result of this vicious cycle, is known as oxidative stress.

Free radicals cause damage by attacking the body's tissue. Free radicals can attack DNA, leading to dysfunction, mutation, and cancer. They can also attack enzymes and proteins, disrupting normal cell activities, or cell membranes, producing a chain reaction of destruction. When free radicals attack lipids (fats), it often results in the formation of plaques within blood vessels, which contributes to improper blood flow, high blood pressure and then increased risk of heart attack and stroke.

While a certain amount of free radicals are formed from the biochemical processes that naturally occur inside the body, if left uncontrolled, the free radicals can quickly overwhelm the body's natural defenses and destroy healthy tissues. In addition, high levels of free radicals will increase the overall acidity of body tissue. All cancer cells thrive in an acidic environment, so if the body is constantly inflamed trying to manage the onslaught of toxicity, the cancer killing immune system becomes depleted. This can cause cancer cells to start to grow in large amounts, especially if oxygen levels are low. Trying to heal any issue while the body is in a state of oxidative stress is like planting fresh seeds in a bed full of weeds and mold; those seeds don't stand a chance. Your practitioner will want to help reduce oxidative stress as a basis for your path to wellness.

Detoxification Organs

The Liver

The liver is the primary organ of the detoxification system. The liver functions much like a filter. When unhealthy chemicals and other toxins are ingested, the liver filters them from the blood and clears them from the body. Despite all the work the liver has to do each day, it has an amazing ability to regenerate itself. In fact, the liver is the only organ that can re-grow itself if a section is cut away. However, when the body has to handle too many toxins on a routine basis, the delicate filters within the liver can become clogged. When the liver becomes clogged, its ability to

Symptoms Associated With Natural Detoxification Dysfunction		
Abnormal metabolism of fats (lipids) leading to:	• Abnormalities in the level of fats in the blood stream e.g. elevated LDL cholesterol and reduced HDL cholesterol and elevated triglycerides. • Arteries blocked with fat, leading to high blood pressure, heart attacks and strokes. • Fatty liver and build-up of fat in other body organs. • Obesity and /or inability to lose weight • Sluggish metabolism	Chronic inflammation due to heavy metal toxicity will cause a rise in cholesterol to protect the brain from toxins. Look for natural ways to reduce LDL through reducing toxicity rather than simply reducing the LDL cholesterol with medications.
External Signs	• Coated tongue • Bad breath • Red palms and soles • Flushed facial appearance or excessive facial blood vessels (capillaries/veins) • Acne, Rosacea • Yellow conjunctiva on the eyes • Red swollen itchy eyes (allergic eyes) • Dark circles under the eyes • Brownish spots and blemishes on the skin (liver spots) • Rashes and itchy skin (pruritis)	Skin problems most likely originate in the intestine, where damage by toxins (including but not limited to heavy metals), non nutritious foods and stress, have damaged the intestinal lining, thus allowing toxins into the system.
Digestive Problems	• Gall stones and gall bladder disease • Intolerance to fatty foods • Intolerance to alcohol • Indigestion • Reflux • Nausea • Abdominal bloating • Constipation • Irritable bowel syndrome • Hemorrhoids	Heavy metals can combine with bile from the gallbladder and cause it to become more alkaline, thus providing an environment that parasites and bacteria enjoy. Parasites can then block up the bile duct so digestive enzymes are not released.
Nervous System	• Depression • Mood changes such as anger and irritability • Poor concentration and "foggy brain" • Overheating • Recurrent headaches associated with nausea	Heavy metals impact neurotransmitter function and nutrient deficiencies.
Immune Dysfunction	• Allergies: sinus, hay fever, asthma, dermatitis, hives, etc. • Skin rashes and inflammations • Chemical and food sensitivities • Autoimmune diseases • Chronic Fatigue Syndrome and Fibromyalgia • Recurrent viral, bacterial and parasitic infections	Free radicals increase leading to chronic inflammation, resulting in a range of chronic conditions.
Blood sugar Problems	• Craving for sugar • Hypoglycemia • Mature onset diabetes is common in those with a fatty liver	Heavy metals, especially mercury, can result in overgrowth of yeast and fungus. Mytotoxins from fungus inhibits the absorption of insulin.
Hormonal Issues	• Intolerance to hormone replacement therapy (e.g. side effects) • Menopausal symptoms such as hot flashes may be more severe • Premenstrual syndrome may be more severe	A blocked gallbladder means less HDL (good) cholesterol is produced so then hormone levels can be affected. Zinc is important for progesterone and testosterone production.
Chronic Fatigue	• Insomnia or excessive sleepiness • Low energy • "Sweatpants and slippers" behavior	Adrenal glands can be weakened by continual inflammatory response. Heavy metals bind to oxygen and hemoglobin in blood, lowering oxygen levels causing lack of energy and increased risk for cancer which thrives on a low-oxygen environment.

clear toxins from the blood is reduced in the same way a clogged air filter on your vacuum cleaner reduces the amount of air that can move through the machine.

The Intestines

After detoxification, the liver redistributes the nutrients into the blood stream. The various chemicals, toxins, drugs, heavy metals and excess sex hormones that were extracted are dumped by the liver into the bile. The bile transports these substances into the small intestine and they continue through the intestinal tract. The final phase of the transformation of toxins takes place in the colon or large intestine. The large intestine is approximately four and a half feet long and is responsible for removing liquid, toxins, and various minerals from the digested food, and for solidifying the stool. If the intestinal passage becomes delayed, for example with constipation, the food that cannot be eliminated ferments and putrefies. The healthy beneficial microorganisms of the intestinal microflora may mutate into aggressive microbes which excrete toxins of their own. Constant irritation of the mucous membranes by toxic metabolites, additives, pesticides, antibiotics, medications, etc., can damage the intestinal mucosa and make it porous.

The Kidneys

The kidneys are so important to bodily functions including the elimination process, that there are two! Blood carries waste products to the kidneys via the renal artery. Inside each kidney, blood is transported to 1.2 million filtering units called nephrons (pronounced NEFF-rons). The cells in nephrons take in the liquid portion of the blood and filter out impurities (urea, mineral salts, and other toxins). Necessary substances such as certain salts, water, glucose (sugar), and other nutrients are returned to the blood stream via the renal vein.

The waste-containing fluid that remains in the nephrons is called urine. Urine is ninety five percent water in which the waste products are dissolved. A pair of tubes called ureters carry urine from the kidneys to the urinary bladder. The bladder is a hollow muscular sac located in the pelvis that is collapsed when empty, but pear-shaped and distended when full. An adult bladder can hold more than sixteen ounces of urine. The bladder empties urine into the urethra, a duct leading to outside the body. A sphincter muscle around the urethra at the base of the bladder controls the flow of urine between the two. As a side note, estrogen depletion can contribute to more urgency, frequency of urination and sometimes result in urinary incontinence.

The volume of urine excreted is controlled by the antidiuretic hormone (ADH), which is released by the pituitary gland. If an individual perspires a lot or fails to drink enough water, special nerve cells in the hypothalamus (a region of the brain controlling body temperature, hunger, and thirst) detect the low water concentration in the blood. They then signal the pituitary gland to release ADH into the blood, where it travels to the kidneys. With ADH present, the kidneys reabsorb more water from the urine and return it to the blood. The volume of urine is thus reduced. On the other hand, if an individual takes in too much water, production of ADH decreases. The kidneys do not reabsorb as much water, and the volume of urine is increased. Alcohol inhibits ADH production and therefore increases the output of urine.

The Lungs

The respiratory tract, the lungs and bronchi, mainly evacuate toxins in the form of carbonic gas and phlegm. Healthy membranes of the alveoli (air sacks) do not let solid waste penetrate. However, due to constant irritation by infectious microbes and other irritants, the alveoli may become porous and act as an emergency exit for toxins that the liver, kidneys and the intestinal tract did not succeed in eliminating. These substances are transported by the blood stream towards the lungs and bronchi, they squeeze through the alveoli and we cough them up as phlegm. This phlegm not only consists of microbes and the products of their activity, but also of waste resulting from insufficient digestion and excretion.

The Skin

The skin is the largest organ in the body. Sometimes the other organs of elimination need help from the skin. Any toxin/waste that is soluble in water can also be eliminated through sweat. If liver, kidneys and lungs do not fulfill the detox tasks sufficiently, the body needs help from the skin. It evacuates the waste products that are classified as crystals through the sweat glands. Crystals are the residues of the metabolism of food rich in protein, such as meat, fish, eggs, dairy products, legumes and cereals. Uric acid and urea are part of the group of crystals. These may also result from an excess of refined sugar or very acidic food. Other types of waste products and toxins are excreted in the form of rashes. If you have eczema or other persistent rashes, it could well be an indication that your body is working hard to detoxify a particular toxicant.

The Lymph System

The lymph system plays a crucial part in detoxification and defense. About two liters of lymph fluid circulate in the lymphatic vessels that cover the body from the tips of the toes to the top of the head. These two liters are formed continually from the extra cellular fluid surrounding each cell in the body. This extra cellular fluid penetrates the membrane of the capillaries (the thinnest vessels), to keep the volume of lymph fluid constant and to allow the waste products to leave the cells and be carried away to the blood stream and evacuated.

The network of lymphatic capillaries leads to bigger lymphatic vessels and finally to the lymphatic glands which are placed in groups all along the lymphatic pathways. The lymph glands have lots of functions related to immunity and purification of the body fluids to maintain its proper functioning. These lymphatic glands are stations where infectious agents are filtered, and lymphocytes (white blood cells, "the defenders") are produced. If the work of the lymph nodes is insufficient, then filtering, degradation, and transport of the waste products will be impeded and the body will be more and more overwhelmed with toxic metabolites and toxins.

Too many toxins in the blood can also affect the functions of other organs. Inadequate detoxification can disrupt the nervous system and brain function which can lead to depression, anxiety, and fatigue. Unhealthy levels of toxins can also cause allergies and skin problems, as well as accelerate the aging process and contribute to degenerative diseases. Constant exposure to toxic chemicals can also contribute to nutritional deficiencies, which can compromise the body's ability to provide anti-oxidant protection. If you are generally a healthy person but find yourself experiencing one or more of the above health issues, it could be a sign that your body's detoxification system isn't functioning properly. The good news is that it is possible to stop the progression of your symptoms and reverse the effects on your health.

Heavy Metals

Some metals/minerals, collectively known as heavy metals because of their "heavy" molecular weight, are known to be toxic to humans. Heavy metal toxicity, just like chemical toxicity, is becoming a very pressing health hazard. Bodies are assailed by chemicals and heavy metals on a daily basis, oftentimes from the most innocent-looking sources, such as cookware or children's toys. Heavy metals like cadmium, lead, mercury, nickel arsenic, aluminum and more are so pervasive in society today, there is no longer a question of whether or not we are toxic, but rather how toxic.

Some heavy metal poisoning is acute and comes from very high dose exposures, and is not where we will focus attention in this chapter. Instead, we will look at how chronic, low level environmental exposures can cause heavy metals to accumulate in tissue and how these levels have been linked to the increased risk of various chronic diseases.

Mercury

Mercury is a naturally occurring element that is found in air, water and soil. Exposure to mercury, even small amounts, may cause serious health problems, and is a threat to the development of the child in utero and early in life. Mercury has toxic effects on the nervous, digestive and immune systems, and on lungs, kidneys, skin and eyes. Mercury is considered by the World Health Organization to be one of the top ten chemicals or groups of chemicals of major public health concern.

People are mainly exposed to methylmercury, an organic compound, when they eat fish and shellfish that contain the compound. Mercury can leach into the body from silver-mercury amalgam fillings, or from other sources, and, because it displaces zinc, will cause symptoms of zinc deficiency such as fatigue, PMS, thyroid problem, loss of smell and taste, macular degeneration (a disease of the retina of the eye), prostate enlargement, rheumatoid arthritis, sterility, or immune suppression, even if there is plenty of zinc available.

Lead

Though lead is found frequently in the environment, it has no known purpose in the body; however, the body will confuse lead with calcium and other essential nutrients. Lead will displace calcium from the body leaving the body deficient in calcium. This biochemical confusion can cause permanent damage to the health of both children and adults.

Children and Lead Exposure

In children, lead is most damaging from birth to age six. Children grow at a very fast rate, building bones, developing stronger muscles and creating many connections in their brains. When lead instead of essential nutrients is "available" to the body to build bones, muscle, and brain connections, permanent harm to health can occur. Even at low levels, lead can be harmful and is associated with:

- Learning disabilities resulting in a decreased intelligence (decreased IQ)
- Attention deficit disorder
- Behavior issues
- Nervous system damage
- Speech and language impairment
- Decreased muscle growth
- Decreased bone growth
- Kidney damage

Adults and Lead Exposure

Lead exposure is also a concern for adults even though growth cycles are complete. Since an adult's body is much larger than a child's body, more lead is needed to cause injury, but the harm lead can do to an adult is very serious. High levels of lead can cause:

- Increased chance of illness during pregnancy
- Harm to a fetus, including brain damage or death
- Fertility problems in both men and women
- High blood pressure
- Digestive issues
- Nerve disorders
- Memory and concentration problems
- Muscle and joint pain

Arsenic

Arsenic is a silver-gray or white-metallic element that occurs naturally in the earth's crust. It is odorless and nearly tasteless. Pure arsenic is rare in the environment, and is usually found combined with one or more other elements, such as oxygen or chlorine. Arsenic is also produced as a by-product from smelting copper, cobalt, and lead. Abandoned uranium mines may contain arsenic in the soil and water. Arsenic compounds are used primarily in wood preservatives; in pesticides, primarily on cotton plants; as alloying, or tempering agents for heavy metals; in the manufacture of certain kinds of glass; in solders; and in medicines (yes, medicines).

Exposure to arsenic can come through breathing in contaminated air at work; breathing in sawdust or smoke from burning wood treated with arsenic; or eating food, drinking water, or breathing air that contains arsenic. Exposure can also come from living in areas near copper or lead smelters, industrialized areas where large quantities of arsenic are disposed of in landfills or hazardous waste sites, or areas with unusually high natural levels of arsenic in rock.

Arsenic is a known poison and is listed as a human carcinogen because it has been shown to:

- Cause skin, lung, bladder, liver, kidney, and prostate cancer
- Increase the risk of damage to a developing fetus
- Cause nausea, vomiting, abnormal heart rhythm
- Decrease production of red and white blood cells
- Impair nerve function
- Damage blood vessels
- Cause skin warts and corns, and red or swelling skin
- Damage the liver and kidneys, cause stomach problems, and cause a darkening of the skin
- Cause a sore throat or irritated lungs after breathing in high levels of arsenic

Cadmium

Cadmium is a soft, malleable, bluish white metal found in zinc ores, and to a much lesser extent, in the cadmium mineral greenockite. Common industrial uses for cadmium today are in batteries, alloys, coatings (electroplating), solar cells, plastic stabilizers, and pigments. Cadmium is generally present in the environment at low levels; however, human activity has greatly increased those levels in the last seventy years. Cadmium can travel long distances from the source of emission through air. It is readily accumulated in many organisms, notably molluscs and crustaceans. Lower concentrations are found in vegetables, cereals and starchy roots (from the soil). Human exposure occurs mainly from consumption of contaminated food, active and passive inhalation of tobacco smoke, and inhalation by workers in the non-ferrous metal industry.

Cadmium interferes with several enzymes, in particular preventing the kidneys from producing a vitamin D-derived hormone that controls calcium levels. When this hormone is not produced, bone minerals are not deposited, and this leads to bone deformities and osteoporosis. Cadmium accumulates primarily in the kidneys and high levels can damage the structure of the kidney. High intake of cadmium can lead to disturbances in calcium metabolism and the formation of kidney stones. Cadmium impacts the respiratory system as well, and has been classified as a human carcinogen.

Aluminum

Aluminum is the most abundant metallic element found on the earth and is present naturally in the air, water and soil. It can be absorbed into the body through the digestive tract, the lungs and the skin, and is also absorbed by, and accumulates in, the body's tissues. It is used in the process of making cooking pots and pans, utensils and foil, indeed today, aluminum is found in almost everything. Just about all foods that need raising agents or additives, such as cakes and biscuits, contain aluminum. Candy frequently contains aluminum-enhanced food coloring. It is in tea, cocoa and malt drinks, in some wines and sodas and in most processed foods. Other items such as over the counter pain killers, anti-inflammatory products, douche preparations, antiperspirants, toothpaste, dental amalgams, bleached flour, grated cheese, table salt, and beer, (especially when the beer is in aluminum cans) also contain aluminum.

Excessive use of antacids is a common cause of aluminum toxicity in America, especially for those who have kidney problems. Many over the counter type antacids contain amounts of aluminum hydroxide that may be too much for the kidneys to handle properly. Add to that exposure to toxic fluoride in city drinking water, which actually increases the body's uptake of aluminum, in addition to all the other health damaging effects it has in and of itself, and it is no wonder that the number of aluminum toxicity symptoms are on the rise.

Even though aluminum is not considered to be a heavy metal like lead, it can be toxic in excessive amounts and even in small amounts if it is deposited in the brain. There is growing evidence that the accumulation of aluminum (which replaces magnesium) in the brain is a risk factor not only for Alzheimer's disease but may also be linked to other neurological conditions such as Parkinson's and Multiple Sclerosis. Other symptoms increasingly associated with excess aluminum exposure include:

• Colic
• Rickets

- Gastrointestinal problems
- Interference with the metabolism of calcium
- Extreme nervousness
- Anemia
- Headaches
- Decreased liver and kidney function
- Memory loss
- Speech problems
- Softening of the bones
- Aching muscles

Aluminum is excreted by the kidneys, therefore toxic amounts can impair kidney function. The brain is normally protected by a blood-brain barrier, which filters the blood before it reaches the brain. Elemental aluminum does not pass through this barrier, but certain compounds of aluminum, such as aluminum fluoride do. Interestingly, many city water supplies are treated with both aluminum sulfate and aluminum fluoride. Unfortunately, these two chemicals can combine easily in the blood and, as aluminum fluoride is poorly excreted in the urine, aluminums builds up in the tissues of the body.

Polychlorinated Biphenyls (PCB's)

PCBs belong to a broad family of man-made organic chemicals known as chlorinated hydrocarbons. PCBs were domestically manufactured from 1929 until their manufacture was banned in 1979 in the United States of America. Many other countries have also banned or severely restricted use of these chemicals. Generally, PCBs are very stable which explains their persistence in the environment. In rivers and lakes, PCBs attach to sediments where they can remain buried for a long time before eventual release into water and air. PCBs in the air can reach the ground with falling rain and snow, or simply when suspended particles settle with gravity. At high temperatures, PCBs can burn and generate dangerous by-products such as dioxins. While PCBs tend not to evaporate or to dissolve easily in water, they are, however, very soluble in fat and similar substances, which explains why PCBs can build up in animal fat, especially oily fish. Thus humans can accumulate PCBs from the food they eat.

Multiple studies have now shown that farmed salmon are likely the most PCB-contaminated protein source in the U.S. food supply. On average, farmed salmon have sixteen times the dioxin-like PCBs found in wild salmon, four times the levels in beef, and three point four times the dioxin-like PCBs found in other seafood. If you are buying fresh fish, especially fatty fish, the healthiest choice is fish that is wild caught, not farmed.

PCBs are known to cause a variety of adverse health effects including cancer in animals. PCBs have also been shown to cause a number of serious non-cancer health effects, including impacts on the immune system, reproductive system, nervous system, and the endocrine system. The different health effects of PCBs may be interrelated, as alterations in one system may have significant implications for the other systems of the body.

Toxic Load

We all know that toxins and toxicants are poisons. We would never think of drinking a cup of coffee laced with rat poison, yet every day we eat, drink, breathe, and touch some very poisonous chemicals. While the body is continually working to detoxify, scientific evidence now indicates that not only is it a struggle for the body to keep up with the need for detoxification, but that toxins also reduce the body's natural ability to detoxify and eliminate toxins. The slow, sneaky, but inevitable imbalance of toxins in vs toxins out, leads to toxic overload – a steady build-up of accumulated toxins and complex chemical mixtures that we are not adequately eliminating. In the last seventy years the number of chemicals created and manufactured has gone through the roof. Back in the 1950's this was exciting, all this science, all this chemistry, making new things and making new things possible. It was some years before evidence that some chemicals can have problem effects began to be accepted. Now it is clear that the rates of chronic disease have grown alongside the number of chemicals manufactured and released into the environment.

More recently, there is a newer theory that an accumulating toxicant burden can lead to hypersensitivity to normal things in the environment. Think about pollen allergies, or dander allergies or any kind of allergy. When a body reaches its limit on toxicants, tolerance for usual things in the environment is no longer possible. We all have friends who come to work with runny noses and red eyes saying through a sneezing fit "it is my allergies". That might even be you!

Working with a practitioner to identify hidden toxicants can be a great place to start understanding how your body is currently functioning. Yes, there are lots of steps you can take right now to begin reducing the number of toxicants added to your body, but if you have high levels of certain toxicants you will need to work with a practitioner to make sure that you don't just simply mobilize toxicants without excreting them from your body. Remember the three phases of detoxification: you need to have all of them working in order to detoxify your body safely. Your practitioner will probably start with an in-depth analysis of the symptoms you are experiencing and a full medical history. Try to have written down as much as you can remember about your history of chronic disease as this will help the practitioner know where to start. Expect to do some heavy metals testing, and also expect that your health insurance plan might not pay for all or any of this or that it is applied to an out of network deductible. Sometimes that is a frightening thought, so get an idea from your practitioner of what the cost of testing will be so you are prepared.

Lab testing available includes the following:

Testing For Toxins - Available Tests Include The Following	
Test Sample Type	**Purpose of the Test**
Adipose Tissue	Analysis of fat tissue for presence of pesticide and solvent residues
Hair	Commonly used to assess heavy metals (although not all individuals excrete metal equally in their hair)
Blood and Serum	Used to assess the physiological effects of toxins
Urine	To test for toxin metabolites
Stool	Can be useful for testing for heavy metals particularly in children
Gene Testing	To identify potential weaknesses in the detoxification process

Once your practitioner has identified the toxins that are harming your body and the ways that your body detoxifies, then you will start on a detoxification treatment protocol that is designed for you, for your situation, and for your body. The Appendix lists a number of laboratories that can provide specialist testing for toxins and toxicants.

Minimize Exposure to Toxins

There are things you can start doing right here, right now to decrease the body's burden of toxins. The first step to minimizing exposure is to raise toxin awareness level by learning to identify the hidden sources of toxins in food, common household products, and the environment. Read labels closely before buying any consumer goods and, when in doubt, err on the side of caution.

With more than one hundred thousand chemicals in common use in North America, it is a constant challenge to limit exposure to these harmful substances in their many forms. It is advisable to choose food sources that are locally and organically grown whenever possible. This will help to greatly reduce exposure to toxic pesticides, herbicides, and fungicides. Purchasing unsprayed, naturally fertilized fruits and vegetables supports sustainable and non-toxic agricultural practices. Reducing some common sources of toxins in and around the home can be as simple as taking off street shoes when we enter the home.

Detoxify While You Eat!

Regularly eating the foods listed below will help reduce your body's toxic load. Always eat organic when you can, and if you can't – wash fruits and vegetables carefully before eating. While you avoid foods that you know or suspect you have intolerance for, here are some suggestions:

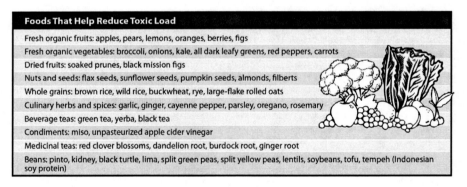

Foods That Help Reduce Toxic Load

Fresh organic fruits: apples, pears, lemons, oranges, berries, figs

Fresh organic vegetables: broccoli, onions, kale, all dark leafy greens, red peppers, carrots

Dried fruits: soaked prunes, black mission figs

Nuts and seeds: flax seeds, sunflower seeds, pumpkin seeds, almonds, filberts

Whole grains: brown rice, wild rice, buckwheat, rye, large-flake rolled oats

Culinary herbs and spices: garlic, ginger, cayenne pepper, parsley, oregano, rosemary

Beverage teas: green tea, yerba, black tea

Condiments: miso, unpasteurized apple cider vinegar

Medicinal teas: red clover blossoms, dandelion root, burdock root, ginger root

Beans: pinto, kidney, black turtle, lima, split green peas, split yellow peas, lentils, soybeans, tofu, tempeh (Indonesian soy protein)

Optimal nutrition is essential when dealing with metal toxicity because if you are deficient in essential metals, your body will use toxic metals as "stand-ins" instead. For example:

- Calcium is replaced by lead which deposits primarily in bone, and disrupts the formation of red blood cells. Lead contributes to poor bone health such as osteopenia and osteoporosis

- Zinc is replaced by cadmium, which tends to accumulate heavily in your kidneys. Deficiencies in zinc can lead to loss of taste, low libido, PMS etc. Cadmium overload is also associated with peripheral neuropathy (nerve disease)

- Magnesium is replaced by aluminum, which, among other things, induces brain chemistry changes and has been identified as a contributing factor to developing Alzheimer's
- Manganese is replaced by nickel, which is carcinogenic
- Iron displacement can lead to anemia
- Copper displacement can lead to anemia, thyroid dysfunction, impaired digestion and scoliosis

Secondly, you also need vital nutrients to aid your natural detoxification process and your practitioner can help you by recommending high quality blended supplements that provide what you need without overdosing you or overwhelming you with too many bottles.

{ Guidelines to Limit Toxic Exposure }

- Use glass, cast iron, carbon steel, titanium, and enamel cookware. Both aluminum and non-stick cookware are well known for their toxic dangers, and stainless steel can expose you to carcinogenic nickel.
- Minimize consumption of restaurant food as restaurants are required to use stainless steel pots and vats.
- Avoid stainless steel thermoses; the glass lined kinds are best.
- Avoid cosmetics with aluminum bases, mineral powders that contain bismuth, and aluminum-laden antiperspirants.
- Avoid vaccinations that inject mercury or aluminum directly into your bloodstream.
- Avoid and remove dental amalgam fillings.
- Avoid costume jewelry if you are sensitive to metals.
- Avoid smoking and second hand smoke as it causes cadmium poisoning.
- Make sure you purchase your natural herbal remedies from a reputable source with strict quality testing.
- Avoid conventional household cleaning products.
- Avoid conventional insecticides and herbicides. Also be very cautious when using the "natural alternative" Borax (boric acid), which can also cause serious health problems, including death.

This chapter gives you a quick overview of the impact that toxins and toxicants can have on health. Adverse reactions between you and the environment that have led to chronic disease are not always obvious but practitioners who are trained in Environmental Medicine are best able to find root causes of symptoms and recommend treatment solutions. There is rarely only one offending toxicant that has resulted in chronic disease. Multiple factors have probably contributed to the disease process over time. Individual susceptibility to environmental agents occurs for a variety of reasons including your genetic code, gender, nutritional status, level of exposures to toxicants, infection, and emotional and physical stress.

It is important to remember that if you are struggling with chronic disease, you did not get to this place overnight and there is no pill or detox smoothie that will make it better in a week or ten days. Please understand that it will take several months, if not longer, to undo any damage from environmental forces. Do know however, that there are some gifted practitioners who are able to help you, if you are committed to helping yourself.

Chapter Six Summary – Toxicity

- Natural production of toxins
- Toxicant sources in the environment
- Stages of detoxification
- Detoxification organs: liver, intestines, kidneys, lungs, skin, lymph
- Symptoms of detoxification dysfunction
- Heavy metal damage: mercury, lead, arsenic, cadmium, aluminum, PCB's
- Toxic load
- Testing for heavy metals and toxicants
- Minimizing exposure
- Using food to detoxify

CHAPTER SEVEN

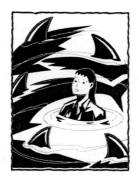

STRESS

If there is one and only one piece of information you take from this chapter – let it be this: too much stress can kill you, or at the very least, make life completely miserable. There are frightening statistics on how much stress the modern person experiences, and mounting evidence that a life lived under prolonged stress harms the body in ways that are profound and long lasting.

Now, don't get me wrong, stressful situations are a natural part of being a creature, any creature, hamster, hyena, heron, or human. The stress response is a triumph of evolution and a necessary part of survival for any species. Traditional human stresses were famine, disease or accidents, threat of harm from a fellow human, attack by a wild animal, separation from the tribe. With the exception of famine, these stressful situations were usually short lived. Take the example of a young hunter out with a couple of other hunters. As he approaches a herd of antelope stealthily moving through the brush, circling upwind, preparing to throw his spear, out of the corner of his eye, he sees a large lion which is also getting close to the antelope. His nerves, already on edge with the focus of the hunt, fire into overdrive as the all-boys bash out in the bush looking for food turns into a potential life or death situation with a hungry lion about to join the party. This sort of situation is natural stress, and the stress response prepares the hunter for fight, freeze or flight. Whatever his decision and subsequent action, his stress response will relax after the hunters either chase off the lion, beat a strategic retreat and let the lion take the field, or get eaten.

We all have experienced sudden stressors in dangerous situations – stepping off a curb and reacting swiftly when a car makes a turn into our path, being approached by an unfamiliar man on the street shouting "hey baby", a teenager losing sight of her cell phone, getting to the checkout stand on the day before Thanksgiving unloading a huge cart of groceries only to discover your wallet has fallen out of your purse and there are twelve people behind you in line sharpening their spears and pointing them in your direction. We recognize the feeling of a sudden stressor and know how the tension feels in the body. What is harder to recognize is how a series of small little stressors begin to build up in the body over time. Take this average day:

- Alarm goes off – woken suddenly out of a deep sleep, shower and head to the kitchen.

- Three children who need breakfast, open the fridge – discover you forgot to get sausages and eggs, damn, it will have to be high carb cereal again for breakfast.

- Leaving the house late you drive fast through traffic and merging onto the freeway a truck suddenly appears over your left shoulder, horn blasting, where the heck did that come from?

- Sliding into your desk and opening your calendar you discover you were supposed to be in a meeting that started five minutes ago.

- The meeting passes and a couple of big tasks get added to your to-do list.

- As lunchtime approaches, your coworker asks if you want to go to lunch, you pass and have another cup of coffee to keep you going.

- A reminder goes off on your calendar that you have to leave early to pick up your daughter to take her to an appointment.

- Weaving through traffic you screech to a halt in front of school and find four text's from her asking where you are. She jumps in and you are off, back in traffic, red lights again, but you get there just four minutes late.

- Then it is home to get dinner before heading out to drive your son to Karate practice.

- You are home by 8pm then it is time to clean up the kitchen after dinner, empty lunch boxes, prepare lunches for the following day, settle the children into bed, put on a load of laundry, open up your personal email. By 10.30 pm the house is quiet and there is finally some time for you to settle down, drink a cup of tea and relax. Your spouse is feeling affectionate but all you have energy for is brushing your teeth and falling into bed.

- Next day – repeat
- Next day – repeat

This doesn't even begin to include the pressure of too many demands on a small family budget, too many distractions and requests for things to buy and things to do, too many comparisons with those that seem to "have it all", trying to be perfect, the stress of aging parents, the stress of dysfunctional family behavior, the stress of constant fear due to family abuse and angry companions, the stress of increasingly demanding work, increasingly busy traffic, increasing number of channels to choose from on TV, increasing numbers of texts and tweets and emails to respond to, increasing amounts of information to try to sort and process.

Days like this are sadly, horribly, very common for many people. With so much to juggle, so much to do, so much to fit in, so many things to remember to do and respond to, the result is a small but insidious increase in small scale stressors that gradually compound over time to form a very stressful life style. And we are not even talking about the big stressors like a death or a divorce or a serious injury.

This chapter will explain how stress affects the body and the mind, and provide some ideas on how you can both reduce the impact of stressful events and also work with a practitioner to heal your body from any current damage due to stress. Let us start by reviewing the biochemistry of a stress response.

Whatever the stressor or threat experienced by someone, the body's response is the same:

1. The autonomic nervous system automatically puts the body and brain on alert.
2. The adrenal gland automatically releases the stress hormone cortisol, and the neurotransmitters norepinephrine (noradrenaline) and epinephrine (adrenaline).
3. The heart automatically beats harder and more rapidly.

4. Breathing automatically becomes more rapid.

5. The thyroid gland automatically stimulates the metabolism.

6. Larger muscles automatically receive more oxygenated blood.

Reread the description of an average busy day above and count all the circumstances that would spike a stress response in you. As you come to the end of the description, observe how you are breathing, are you calm and breathing deeply or has your breath moved to smaller shallower bursts?

Rushing continually from one event to another eventually runs the risk that the autonomic systems are on permanent alert. In the beginning, this can result in gradually increasing levels of circulating cortisol. While this can turn an average person into a superhero in the short term, persistent, sustained stress and demand on the adrenal glands will eventually result in a significant drop in the level of cortisol produced. In effect, the adrenal glands "give up" responding to every stressor and become dysfunctional.

Adrenal Dysfunction

The adrenal glands sit right on top of your kidneys and produce the hormones cortisol, DHEA, and the neurotransmitters norepinephrine and epinephrine. In addition, the adrenal glands also secrete aldosterone, which plays a role in blood pressure regulation and mineral and water resorption in the kidneys. There are three states of adrenal dysfunction:

It is possible to remain in one stage, or progress through each of the stages, or find ways to recover and rebalance from any stage. The key is to be aware of this progression and know that there are solutions.

Symptoms of Adrenal Dysfunction include:

- Stress
- Morning Fatigue
- Difficulty Sleeping
- Decreased Stamina
- Anxiousness
- Irritability
- Nervousness

- Fibromyalgia
- Allergies
- Headaches
- Sugar Cravings
- Dizzy Spells

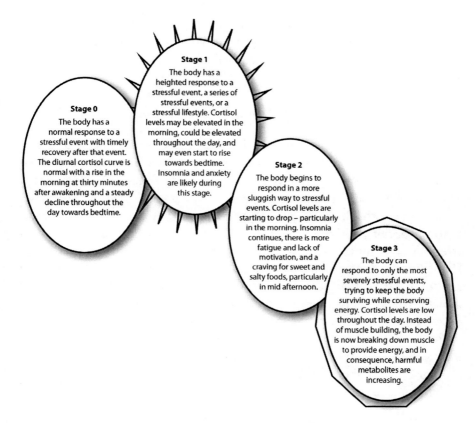

Stage 0

The body has a normal response to a stressful event with timely recovery after that event. The diurnal cortisol curve is normal with a rise in the morning at thirty minutes after awakening and a steady decline throughout the day towards bedtime.

Stage 1

The body has a heighted response to a stressful event, a series of stressful events, or a stressful lifestyle. Cortisol levels may be elevated in the morning, could be elevated throughout the day, and may even start to rise towards bedtime. Insomnia and anxiety are likely during this stage.

Stage 2

The body begins to respond in a more sluggish way to stressful events. Cortisol levels are starting to drop – particularly in the morning. Insomnia continues, there is more fatigue and lack of motivation, and a craving for sweet and salty foods, particularly in mid afternoon.

Stage 3

The body can respond to only the most severely stressful events, trying to keep the body surviving while conserving energy. Cortisol levels are low throughout the day. Instead of muscle building, the body is now breaking down muscle to provide energy, and in consequence, harmful metabolites are increasing.

What is interesting is that the symptoms listed above can be experienced in any of stages one, two, or three, and yet the treatment for each of those stages is different. That is why it is vital to have your practitioner test your adrenal function through salivary hormone testing to determine what your cortisol and DHEA levels are and therefore what would be the best treatment protocol for you.

If you are one of the millions of people experiencing adrenal dysfunction, feeling fatigued and washed up/out is certainly an inconvenience, but there are also some more profound and potentially dangerous changes going on. While much research in the last sixty years has expanded the understanding of the stress response, essentially the way the body responds to just about every stressor there is – real or imagined – has stayed the same. Conditions that contribute to sustained elevated cortisol levels can include stressful lifestyle, anorexia nervosa, obsessive-compulsive disorder, panic disorder, chronic alcoholism, excessive exercising, childhood sexual abuse, living in a dangerous situation because of war or abuse, and depression.

Sources of acute stress are usually fairly obvious, but if you are unsure where your sources of stress come from, your practitioner can help you identify your unique source(s) of chronic stress and their contribution to a chronic health condition.

Consequences of Prolonged Elevated Cortisol

Although the initial stages of the stress response are intended to promote survival, chronic exposure to stressors may lead to periods of elevated cortisol levels that are not reduced appropriately by negative feedback loop. The immune system is one of the primary systems affected by high cortisol. One of cortisol's roles is to suppress the immune system in the short term – especially at the cell level. This is why, when we are under continual stress, it is so much easier to catch a cold, or a series of repeated colds. Remember that cytokines (signaling proteins) are essential in maintaining health and preventing disease, specifically with the body's responses to infection, immune responses, inflammation, trauma, sepsis, cancer, and reproduction. Cortisol reduces some cytokine production resulting in loss of tissues important in immunity, and contributing to increased susceptibility to infection. Additionally, prolonged high cortisol levels may actually be the cause, rather than the consequence, of development or continuation of autoimmune diseases.

Prolonged stress also hinders the non-essential functions of growth and reproduction, including the manufacture of steroid hormones. Stress-induced growth hormone deficiencies have been shown to cause delayed puberty, irregular ovulation and spontaneous abortion in women; and reduced testosterone levels, lower sperm counts and decreased libido in men.

Cortisol increases insulin levels; and as these two hormones rise, fat deposits increase around the middle. Stomach (visceral) fat has abundant cortisol receptors and is very sensitive to the effects of cortisol and insulin. It is a vicious circle, the fat cells around the tummy have lots of receptors the end up attracting more fat, (think flash mob fat around your stomach). This vicious cycle inevitably plays a role in the development of such diseases as insulin resistance, hyperlipidemia (high lipids/triglycerides), cardiovascular disease, and hypertension.

In addition, increases in cortisol-induced abdominal fat are associated with an increase in both free radicals (from oxidative stress) and in the number of inflammatory cytokines. Oxidative stress is made worse with the absence of protective hormones. For example, stress-induced elevations of cortisol and reductions in the brain-protective hormones

DHEA and estrogen, result in more oxidative stress and increased nerve cell death. As the number of free radicals go up the need for detoxification increases, and yet continual stress means the detoxification process can't keep up with all toxins. In fact, stress-induced high cortisol and its cardiovascular effects increase the mortality risk by two to three times, and decrease life expectancy by several years. Yes – stress can kill you!

The Other Side of the Coin – Low Cortisol

Low cortisol, called hypocortisolism, applies to any condition in which levels of cortisol are significantly lower than are expected. Evidence suggests that low cortisol may be a common, yet under-evaluated, consequence of exposure to severe acute stress and chronic intermittent stress. Studies have confirmed states of low cortisol in people frequently exposed to stressful environments, those with unpredictable schedules, and in those with traumatic early life experiences. Low cortisol levels can have a profound impact on inflammation. Cortisol is a natural anti-inflammatory agent. Without cortisol, inflammation has a greater chance of running rampant in the body. There is a strong correlation between low cortisol levels and chronic inflammatory states such as fibromyalgia, rheumatoid arthritis, irritable bowel syndrome, food intolerances, and more.

Testing Cortisol Levels

Most healthcare practitioners are moving towards measuring cortisol levels in saliva at four different times during the day. These measurements are then plotted onto a graph which shows the pattern of your cortisol levels over the day. Here again is the diagram below shows ideal cortisol patterns.

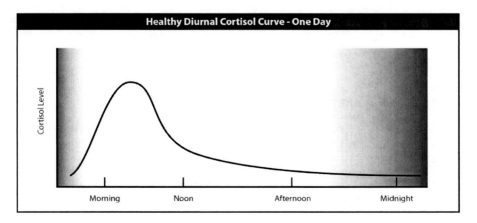

There are a few reasons that practitioners are now using saliva testing rather than serum or urine testing. First – spitting into a tube, at home, is far easier than getting a blood draw at a lab four times a day. Second, blood tests are really good at identifying more serious disease states, but not as good at identifying less severe, but still very debilitating dysfunctional states. Why wait until you get to a severe disease state to do something? Just by the fact that you are reading this book and looking for answers means you don't want to get to that point - you want guidance and support to start back on a path to wellness now.

All practitioners are familiar with Cushings Syndrome (which describes a set of symptoms related to continually very high cortisol levels) and Addison's Disease, (a rare, chronic condition where the adrenal gland does not produce enough cortisol), but fewer practitioners are familiar with the concept of adrenal dysfunction. When looking for a practitioner to work with you, you will want to find out what they know about helping patients with Chronic Fatigue and Adrenal Dysfunction.

Summary of Stress and its impact on the body

1. Metabolic/Glycemic Regulation

When the brain perceives stress, its main focus is to ensure that there is enough glucose (blood sugar) to make sure the brain and the muscles can operate as needed. One of cortisol's roles is to help make sure that this glucose supply is adequate by stimulating gluconeogenesis (the making of glucose). Cortisol will also increase insulin resistance in areas of the body that are not essential to survival. While this function is essential for fight or flight, problems occur if there is too much or too little circulating glucose. When chronic overproduction of cortisol and insulin has resulted in increased belly fat, we also know that the belly fat itself will escalate the number of inflammatory messengers that will then perpetuate the vicious cycle by raising cortisol. Ugh!

2. Inflammation

To repeat (probably ad nauseam by this stage in the book), cortisol is an important anti-inflammatory agent. As discussed in the Chapter on Pain, when there is any inflammation in the body – either through injury or toxic substance, cortisol is produced as part of the response to manage that foreign substance. Maintaining healthy and optimal levels of cortisol is important for managing the body's response to inflammation. An immune system that is in great condition will only be minimally affected by small causes of stress. On the other hand, even small causes of stress can be too much for a weakened immune system.

3. Heart Health

Stress raises the heart rate and so can strain the circulatory system. Stress also elevates blood cholesterol levels, while epinephrine (adrenaline) and norepinephrine (noradrenaline) increase the production of free fatty acids. Hypertension (consistently raised blood pressure over several weeks) is a major risk factor in coronary heart disease (CHD). However, CHD may also be caused by eating too much salt, drinking too much coffee or alcohol (which are common coping behaviors in response to stress).

4. Sleep Disorders

You may remember from the Chapter on Sleep that during slow-wave sleep, cortisol release is normally suppressed and there should be a rise in melatonin and growth hormone secretion at this time. Exposure to chronic stressors disrupts this normal diurnal pattern. The result can be a rise in cortisol levels in the evening hours and during initial phases of sleep. An elevated level of cortisol at night can cause sleep fragmentation, raising cortisol levels even further. Insomnia and depression are common in this situation. Sleep apnea can disrupt the release of cortisol and other adrenal hormones and can also promote the development of secondary metabolic syndrome, hypertension, and inflammatory diseases.

5. Mental and Emotional

Non-physical events such as grief, excitement, fear, anxiety, guilt, embarrassment, all can trigger a robust stress response. Similarly, events such as public speaking, performance evaluations, sky diving or dental appointments will increase cortisol in many people. Research has shown that the magnitude of the response and recovery to these stressors is based on the individual's perception rather than the stressors themselves. The four key factors that determine the magnitude of the response to a mental/emotional stressor are:

a) how new the experience is

b) how unpredictable the experience is

c) what threat there is to body or ego

d) sense of loss of control

Individual characteristics of the person are also relevant – age, gender, and hereditary predisposition, coupled with personality characteristics (i.e. introversion and low self-esteem), and prenatal and early childhood experiences.

6. Digestive

Stress responses have an effect on the digestive system. During stress, digestion is slowed and can completely stop. This may affect the health of the digestive system and cause ulcers, inflammatory bowel disorder, poor absorption of nutrients, and gut permeability. Adrenaline released during a stress response may also contribute to ulceration and slow healing from existing ulcers.

7. Memory

The hippocampus is a section of the brain focused on learning and memory and it turns out that stress hormones have a fondness for the cells in the hippocampus. This "attraction" is a problem because stress hormones can dismantle the networks in the brain that store memories and can also significantly reduce the hippocampus's capacity to form new neurons and therefore new memories. Too much stress, or one extreme acute stressful event can, literally, make it impossible to learn or recall the incident.

8. Allergies

Springtime brings us sunshine, flowers, and unfortunately for more than sixty million people in the United States, seasonal allergies. Allergic disorders, including asthma, allergic rhinitis and eczema, are widely considered to be rising in prevalence at epidemic rates. Allergies are an abnormal immune reaction. The human immune system is designed to protect the body from potential harm and in people who have allergies, the immune system will react to allergens (substances that trigger an immune response). These allergens can be food, pollen, plants, water contaminants, tobacco smoke, pesticides, heavy metals, pet and pest dander, infectious agents (viruses, molds), and stress.

The immune system will produce immunoglobulin E, (IgE), antibodies for each allergen. The antibodies will cause cells in the body to produce histamines. These histamines will act on different areas of the body (eyes, throat, nose, gastrointestinal tract, skin or lungs) to produce symptoms of an allergic reaction: redness, swelling, sneezing, runny nose, red eyes, irritation, and so on. Once this cascade of immune dys-regulation is triggered, allergic symptoms often develop and multiply. Sometimes known as the "allergic march" once you develop one allergic trait (e.g. eczema), others are likely to follow.

Many studies show that the nervous and immune systems, are closely linked. This link has even given rise to a new field of study called psychoneuroimmunology. Practitioners now know that when the body is under stress it feels threatened and produces brain chemicals and hormones that trigger the immune system. Excessive psychological stress and allergy disorder have been linked together in clinical practice for centuries. Many allergic conditions have long been considered psycho-somatic disorders which had worsened outcomes for people with high levels of psychosocial stress. If your allergies have been getting worse over time, or there seem to be more and more things that you have an allergic response to, then stress could be a significant factor.

Stress in the Modern Environment

The next section of this chapter will pay attention to the ways in which modern life in the twenty first century has impacted stress levels for millions of people. If we try to define stress, it is really quite hard to do so. Driving through snow in a small, aging car may bring on fears of imminent death for one person, while another can simply put on the tire chains and drive merrily on whistling happily. Managing with limited finances can give one person an ulcer, while another finds ways to be resourceful and see abundance in the simple joy of being human. Trying to define stress by looking at how the body behaves is also not much help, the aroused state of awareness experienced when facing a loud angry, barking dog is not that much different from the aroused state of awareness while having sex, because an aroused state is common to both frightening and pleasurable situations.

Stress can be thought of as a psycho-physiological process that results from both the appraisal of a given situation to assess potential adversity <u>and</u> the ability (either perceived or actual) to cope with that potentially adverse situation. Situations can be experiences in daily life, including daily hassles (ordinary stressors from interactions with family, neighbors and/or school/in the work place) as well as major life events, which may be either positive or negative, such as a large promotion that requires significantly increased physical and mental effort, or losing one's job resulting in financial crisis. Based on their duration, stressors are often considered:

- acute (minutes to hours)
- sub-acute (less than one month duration)
- chronic (months to years)

Intensity of the stress, even when acute, may have longer lasting effects that can overlap with a less intense stressor lasting for a prolonged period of time. For example – loss of a spouse can overlap with the ongoing stress of single parenting. Further, repetitive acute stressors (the same ones or even different ones) may, with time and intensity, have similar effects to that of a single long term stressor.

Hans Selye, the first major researcher to focus on stress, defined stress as "the non-specific responses of the body to any demand for change." The key words could well be *"any demand for change"*. For most people – being in the presence of a loud, angry, barking dog is not a comfortable situation – it creates feelings of fear of harm (being bitten or worse). Most people will want the situation to be changed: i.e. – no loud, angry, potentially threatening barking dog anywhere near them.

Another example could be driving from one location to another. Leaving with twenty five minutes to do a twenty minute drive but hitting a tailback in traffic that turns the drive into forty minutes, will often make the driver wish things were different ("I should have left earlier, I should have picked the surface street route, I want all other cars in the known universe vaporized", and so on). The driver wishes for an open road and a smooth trip to make the appointment on time. The difference between what was wanted/anticipated and what actually happened is where there is the potential for feelings of stress.

Continuing this theme, here are some more examples in varying degrees of severity that illustrate the difference between what was anticipated/expected and what was the reality.

In some of the situations above the stress is real, in others the stress is imagined and, unfortunately, humans can generate the same response simply by *anticipating* stress, whether or not it occurs, and whether or not it is merited. Driving through traffic to an appointment may bring

Stress... Expectations vs. Reality	
What Was Anticipated/Expected	**What Happened**
The promotion and increased pay	No promotion, same pay, same tight budget
Quiet walk home	A speeding car mounted the curb right by you missing you by five feet.
Time to respond to the list of questions provided by your boss last week.	Coworker was out so you had to pick up their work as well as finish your own, but in the same amount of time.
Long, happy loving marriage	Abuse followed by divorce
Love and acceptance from parents	Absent mother and reserved father
Living a normal life with family	Residential area suddenly becomes part of a war zone
Plenty of time to cook the 14 pound fresh turkey for Thanksgiving	The turkey was put in the freezer by mistake and is completely solid and the guests will be here in 4 hours.
Comfortable win in a basketball game with a 10 point difference.	Being on the line to make the foul shot to win the game
Stay in the same school all the way through High School with familiarity and friends	Having to move to a new town and meet a whole bunch of new kids, repeatedly
Wanting to be able to pay the bills, have enough to eat and save for a vacation	Water heater broke and needs replacing and installing, can't save this month.

up old fears of getting into trouble for being late, wasting other people's time, missing out, seeming a fool, not getting a parking place, wasting money, and so on. Such internal chitter chatter in the brain unnecessarily saps energy and increases tension, and all over something that might be completely false.

How much control someone has over a situation has a profound influence over how stressful a particular experience will be. Research done by psychologist Martin Seligman led to him developing the term "learned helplessness". In learned helplessness studies, an animal is repeatedly exposed to an aversive stimulus from which it cannot escape. Eventually, the animal stops trying to avoid the stimulus and behaves as if it is helpless to change the situation. When opportunities to escape become available, learned helplessness means the animal does not take any action. Learned helplessness results from being trained to be locked into a system. The system may be a family, a community, a relationship, a culture, a tradition, a profession or an institution. Learned helplessness is conditioned behavior in which an individual gives up trying to escape a painful situation after repeatedly failing to escape. We all know that women will often stay in abusive situations when common sense and a sense of self-preservation should suggest that they get the heck out of there. Learned helplessness is why they stay, and lack of control over a situation has a huge impact on the amount of stress experienced by the individual. Learned helplessness can also develop for children. When stuck in a dysfunctional home situation, where there is constant conflict, anger, abuse, criticism, disruption, and bullying, a child frequently has to put up with the situation, having no options to go anywhere else. The combination of the stressful environment and lack of choice are a double whammy to the brain. Teachers frequently observe the grades of star pupils suddenly declining, and later discover changes outside of school such as a bitter divorce in the family.

Stressful Events Analysis

Take a moment here to write out a list of all the things (at least ten) that have caused you stress in the last week. As you write the list - make a note of how your mind and body responds as you recall the stressful incidents. If you find your body beginning to tense up, or you develop a feeling of overwhelm, or sense of lack of control - then keep writing the list, but breathe deeply from your belly at the same time. When you have your list written, next to each item, identify if you had no, some, or a lot of control over the situation. In a third column, rate the events on how stressful each was - high stress, medium or low stress.

Examples of Stressful Circumstances				
Stressful Circumstance	Degree of Control	Level of Stress	What is the story you are writing in your head about the situation?	In the big scheme of things, is this life threatening?
Ending of a love affair	Medium	Medium	I feel unlovable, I don't belong, I don't have a tribe to belong to	Not really (but it can feel like it)
Work load increasing out of proportion to the amount of time available	None	High	I HAVE to get all of this done in order to keep people happy, especially my boss	No
Expected delivery for a key business meeting is lost	None	Medium	I am going to be held accountable for this even though it isn't my error	No
Late for a doctor's appointment	High	High	I am a terrible person I should have planned my time better, now I am going to waste her time	No
Hood flew up on my car while driving	None	High	Holy cow, I could have crashed and died	Yes
Gutter broke leaving rain water cascading down the front of the house	Medium	High	Now I have one more thing to do, and it's urgent, I have to make sure the water doesn't seep into the house	No

Life situations can create stress for several reasons:

1. We feel unprepared for them

2. We are unhappy about them

3. We don't feel able to cope with them

Now go back through your list and categorize each of the stressful events into the three categories here. There is a simple point to this exercise which is to allow yourself to become aware of the types of things that you find stressful, and to give some thought to the messages and stories you play over and over in your own mind that perpetuate the feelings of stress.

Many times we create our own stress because of faulty perceptions about a situation. These faulty perceptions are things we can learn to correct. While it is hard to agree on a specific definition of stress, consistent clinical research confirms that the sense of having little or no control is always distressful – and that is what stress is all about. So if stress is about being in a situation where you feel you have little control, how can you begin to change that?

Someone once said to me that feeling stressed and out of control was like sitting on the tail of a dragon as it flew through the air, there was no way to have any control, all that could be done was to simply hang on. For many, many people this is probably a very applicable description of how they feel about their lives.

One of the most important steps you can take in returning your body to health, is to start working on how to climb along the tail of the dragon so that you have it harnessed and you are in charge. I like that analogy because I love the idea of being able to soar through the air in charge of my destiny, a smile on my face, wearing a T shirt that says "Dragon Tamer Extraordinaire."

Taming Your Dragon

None of what is written below will be very new to you, there is plenty of information available to help you with each of these ideas, what I am hoping is now that you understand the biochemistry of how your body works, you can review these ideas in a new light and decide which approaches you can incorporate into your life as you work with your practitioner to rebalance your body and mind.

Learn Relaxation Techniques

Practicing meditation or breathing awareness every day can relieve chronic stress and realign your outlook in a more positive way. Good breathing habits alone can improve both your psychological and physical well-being. Think back – no matter how far back you have to go – to a time where you lay down on your back and just relaxed. Maybe it was in your yard under a shady tree on a hot summer day, or on a beach, or in a mountain meadow, maybe it was on your sofa, with music playing in the background. For many people, it was long ago, before the realities of being grown up with responsibilities and to-do lists and jobs and children crowded in. Wherever it was, go to that place in your mind if you can. At that time, laid down on your back, eyes closed or looking up, you would have been breathing deeply from your belly; big long slow breaths that filled your lungs and led you to a place of calm and relaxation. When you lie on your back it is almost impossible not to breathe deeply from your belly. Just as short breaths from the top of your lungs signal stress to your brain, those deep belly breaths tell your brain that "Everything is Okay". Although you might get funny looks if you do this, when you find yourself in a stressful situation and are breathing shallowly from the top of your lungs, lie down. Find a way to lie down on the floor for five to ten minutes and breathe deeply. If you absolutely can't lie down, then place your hands over your belly and actively breathe deeply for as long as you can. Not just until you count to ten, although that is often a useful tool when communicating with teenagers, but longer, until your brain gets the message "it is all good, nothing to see here, move it along." Learn to recognize if you are churning something from the past or fussing about something in the future, for if you are locked in the past or living in the future you do not have any free energy to heal in the moment.

Set Realistic Goals

Learning to say "No" is essential for some people. Assess your schedule and identify tasks or activities that you can or should let go. Don't automatically volunteer to do something until you've considered whether it is feasible and healthy for you to do so. There is an amazing study that looked at AIDS patients and how they fared over the duration of their illness. There was one characteristic that differentiated those who survived longer, it was the capacity to say "no" to a favor.

As we have discussed before, you must first put on your own mask before you can help another. That doesn't mean you are selfish, far from, it means that you value yourself enough to take care of yourself first. This can be a real challenge for people who are people-pleasers. For such people (and you know if you are one of them) saying "yes" is a habit, and may even be an addiction because it makes them feel as if they are important and as if they are contributing to a cause. The drawback with this perpetual "yessing" is that the search for validation is coming from outside rather than from inside. Perpetual "yessers" usually lack confidence and they worry how others will view them when they say "no". But saying yes too often can make you sick. If you are over-committed you will get less sleep, and be more likely to be juggling multiple priorities (thus causing stress), churning things in your brain and maybe becoming depressed because you feel like a failure when you can't do it all.

One of my favorite quotes is from Hart Moss. "All the mistakes I ever made were when I wanted to say 'No' and said 'Yes'." The skill is in learning how to say "no" nicely, so that you feel comfortable that you haven't destroyed a relationship. There are plenty of ideas on the internet but here are a few guidelines:

- **Be polite but firm.** This shows that while you're sympathetic, your mind is made up. Being wishy-washy only builds false hopes

- **Keep your answer short.** A lengthy justification of why you can't isn't necessary. Try "I'm sorry, I'm not available then" or "I have another commitment"

- **When in doubt, say "no" now and then change your mind later.** It is more disappointing all round if someone is counting on you and then you let them down

Exercise

You don't have to train for a marathon, but regular, moderate exercise helps ease tension and improves sleep and self-esteem. Making exercise a habit is key. Working out is uncomfortable and difficult when you aren't in shape. But the good news is that you don't need to become a complete exercise junkie to get to a place where exercise is no longer a pain. Just like learning to cook, once you reach a minimum proficiency level – in this case fitness level – exercise stops feeling bad and starts feeling good. And just as with cooking healthily, the only way to get there is to start. Your exercise program isn't necessarily about losing weight, it should be about getting the right biochemistry going again, restarting the engines on your heart, on your muscles, on your immune system. Starting exercise can be really difficult if you are experiencing chronic pain, (believe me I know), but even if all you can do is walk to the end of the street (and back), or walk up and down your stairs for ten minutes, or do some stretching while watching a yoga YouTube video, do something. And find a buddy and make a joint commitment to each other to not let each other down. Even if you feel like letting yourself down, if you have made a commitment to an exercise buddy, it is harder to let them down.

Enjoy Yourself

Taking the time for a favorite hobby is a great way of connecting with and nurturing your creative self. Whatever it may be, value yourself by setting aside an evening or even an hour a week to do something you really enjoy. I love to carve wood and to sew and to read and to dance, to hike, to paddle my kayak, to build things, to write. In fact, I have so many things that I love to do, I find it hard to find the time to do them all often enough. But I always do something each day that I truly enjoy, even if it is only for fifteen minutes.

Visualization

Athletes achieve results by picturing themselves crossing the finish line first. Use the same technique to practice "seeing" yourself succeed in whatever situation is uppermost in your mind. There are lots of resources on the internet about visualization, about imagining what you want. The key is to focus on asking for what you want more of. If you have some love in your life, ask for more of that. If you have some money in your life, ask for more of it. If you want to have a particular career path, focus on building on your current skills to move towards what is next for you. Focus on what you want more of rather than on what you don't have. This is tricky with time, something we all wish we had more of. At one point I found myself thinking "I wish I had more time for all the things I want to do", and then I caught myself and added "and I would still like to be employed in my current job". Just the act of asking for more time made me focus on what was important. I didn't want to create more time by losing my job! I wanted to create more time by focusing on what was important to me and cutting out the things that distracted me from my goals. The year I built a cabin in my yard, I found time; I don't quite know how I did, but somehow I found the time to do it. I visualized the cabin, me sitting in it, reading and writing, cat on my keyboard. I kept that image in my mind through all the construction steps. I mean it, I held that vision in my mind at all times, and now I have this lovely little cabin in my yard and the cat loves it!

Maintain a Healthy Lifestyle

As we have talked about in the Chapter on Nutrition, a good diet is often the first thing to go flying out the window when we're feeling stressed. Grabbing quick food loaded with things we'd do better not to eat is often driven by brain chemistry that is on overload. Making a meal instead of buying one ready-made may seem like a challenge, but it will be probably cheaper and certainly better for you, with the added bonus that the simple action of doing something good for yourself can soothe stressful feelings. Aim for low glycemic foods that are as natural as possible. Avoid soda completely, and carry protein based snacks like nuts with you at all times so that you don't end up eating sugary snacks. Your practitioner will be able to recommend some really well balanced protein bars that are a great option to carry around. Avoid sugar like it is anthrax. Remember that the brain doesn't have an "off" button for sugar and it is therefore just so much easier not to start. Remember to separate eating from stress. If you are feeling stressed, your body cannot digest food properly. When you are ready to eat, take a moment to be still, put aside what worries you and instead relish the food in front of you and allow it to nourish you.

Talk About It

Sharing your troubles with a friend may help you to put things in perspective and to feel that you're not alone. You may also learn some other ways to manage stress effectively. Women in particular have sat and connected through talking for millennia. Sitting, chatting and talking is how we bond and build relationships and support each other. Choose your friends wisely though. Invite around you the people who will help support you as you help yourself. If you find you have people around you who put you down for wanting to change, or who dismiss you and your goals, give some hard thought as to whether you want to continue inviting that kind of negative energy into your life. You are going to have a bit of an uphill battle to undo some of your patterns, so you will do best with people who are on your side to support you, who will bring you apple slices instead of donuts, who will validate your feelings rather than dismiss them, who will be proud of you for the changes you want to make, who will be your cheerleaders.

This chapter started with the words "too much stress can kill you, or at the very least, make life completely miserable". This chapter comes later in the book because all the information in the other chapters leads up to this point. Poor sleep, imbalanced hormones, inadequate nutrition, pain and inflammation, high toxic load and lack of exercise all contribute to stress on the body and mind. By now you know that there are a lot of things that you can do to improve your health, feel better, think better, be kinder, be happier, be more productive, whatever it is that you want for yourself. Working in partnership with your practitioner you can undo the impacts of stress and find a new, positive way to be healthy in the world.

Chapter Seven Summary – Stress

- Stress can kill you
- The power house – the adrenal glands
- Role of the stress response
- Modern day stress
- Biology of persistently elevated cortisol levels
- Biology of chronically low cortisol levels
- Testing cortisol levels and adrenal function
- Impact of stress on metabolism, heart, sleep, emotions, digestion, toxicity, allergies
- Real vs perceived stress
- Tools for managing stress: saying No, exercise, visualization, healthy lifestyle

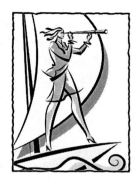

CHAPTER EIGHT

READINESS FOR CHANGE

By making it this far, you have now learned about some important biochemistry that impacts how your body and mind feel. You have also learned that there are lots of things that you can do to move away from the place you are currently at. You could be in any number of places:

- generally feeling well, but wanting to make sure you stay well as you get older;

- feeling tired all the time;

- dealing with persistent symptoms that won't go away for long;

- living with cravings that seem to control you despite your best efforts;

- living with chronic pain and chronic dis-ease of the body.

Wherever you are on your health journey, this final chapter is about supporting your conversation with yourself regarding what you are prepared to do next.

There are many ways that the body will alert the mind to the need to pay attention. We tend to think of pain as something bad, that cancer is bad. But when there is pain or dis-ease of any kind, these are beautiful indicators that something is out of balance and that it might be a good idea to pay attention, look for the underlying root cause, and then do something about it. Structural injuries are simple – it is easy to see that the impact of slipping down a step and hitting the ground hard is the root cause of that torn ligament in a knee. With chronic pain, the challenge is to find those hidden sources of pain and dis-ease.

This book has been all about giving you information and ideas about how to work with a practitioner who can help you get back in balance. It is vital however, to understand that the practitioner you find to work with is neither a magician, nor a miracle worker. Your practitioner has trained and studied to learn how the body works and where it can go wrong. Your practitioner can spend time with you, diagnose some health issues and provide treatment protocols for you to implement. And yet it is You who will be implementing those recommendations, You who will be choosing to step into a healthful state, it is *You* who will be doing the work.

Research has shown that people who successfully change their behavior go through a series of several stages of change, and it is not unusual for them to cycle through these stages three to four times. It is important to recognize where you are in the cycle of change, so you can set appropriate goals and action steps. According to James O. Prochaska, the psychologist who identified the cycles of change, each stage requires different strategies or tools. If you set goals that you are not ready for, you set yourself up for failure. Similarly, if you choose goals that you have already mastered, you will delay your progress. But if you match your goals to your stage of change, you will maximize your ability to effect change.

These are the stages of change:

Stage One: Precontemplation

Individuals in the precontemplation stage of change are not even thinking about changing their behavior. They may not see their choices or their poor state of health as a problem, or they think that others who point out any problems are exaggerating. There are four reasons to be in precontemplation summarized as: reluctance, rebellion, resignation and rationalization.

- Reluctant precontemplators are those who, through lack of knowledge or inertia, do not want to consider change. The impact of the problem has not become fully conscious.

- Rebellious precontemplators have a heavy investment in staying right where they are and in making their own decisions. They are resistant to being told what to do.

- Resigned precontemplators have given up hope about the possibility of change and seem overwhelmed by their health problems.

- Rationalizing precontemplators have all the answers; they have plenty of reasons why their health is not really a problem.

Stage Two: Contemplation

During the contemplation stage, people are ambivalent about changing. Giving up an enjoyed behavior causes them to feel a sense of loss despite the perceived gain. During this stage, people assess barriers (e.g., time, expense, lack of support, lack of self faith, hassle, fear, "I know I need to, but ...") as well as the benefits of change.

Stage Three: Preparation

In this stage, people actually begin to look into what steps they could take to make the change. They gather information about what resources are available and what changes they could make. Having support at this stage is essential. Support and encouragement exponentially increases the chance of success. During this stage people test the waters to see what it could be like to make the needed changes. People try small steps, like taking twenty minutes of exercise every other day, or going to bed and not turning on the television in the bedroom but reading a book instead, or deciding to have a cup of chamomile tea at the end of the day rather than a glass of wine. Some people enjoy the challenge of this stage and the action it begins to call forth, others fear the depth of the impending changes. People who cut the preparation stage short lower their chances of success. It is important to develop a firm, detailed plan of action to follow and reinforce resolutions.

Stage Four: Action

The action stage applies to those people who have made real and overt changes or modifications to their lives and are starting to live their 'new' life with new behaviors. While the chances of relapse and temptation into old patterns are still very strong, there is also openness to receiving help and support. This stage is the 'willpower' stage and short-term rewards to sustain motivation are commonly used. A gym membership might be bought, dark blackout blinds might be installed in the bedroom and the TV removed, a weekly delivery of fresh veg-etables, or a supplement protocol to restore nutritional health is es-tablished so that restoring nutritional health may be started. People are also prone to analyze any behavior changes to enhance their self-confidence and to help make better plans to deal with either per-sonal or external pressures. It is important to realize that, while the action stage is the one that usually receives the most amount of recogni-tion, it is not the only stage during which a person can make progress.

Stage Five: Maintenance

In the maintenance stage, people consolidate the gains made in the action stage and work to prevent relapses. This stage is a long, ongoing, and a critically important process. We all know someone who lost many pounds on a diet, but regained them all in a few months. Successful main-tenance requires active alertness. By this stage, people are working to con-solidate any changes in their behavior, to maintain the 'new' status quo and to prevent relapse or temptation. The former behavior is now seen as no longer desirable and a number of coping strategies have been put in place and are working. In this stage people need to be patient and avoid personal and environmental temptations. Control is shown when shopping at the grocery store because they know it's far easier to not eat a bag of chips if you don't buy it in the first place. There is a need for them to remind them-selves of the progress that has been made already and to stay on the course of change. The risk of lapsing is substantially less than in earlier stages.

Stage Six: Termination

The sixth and final termination stage, is the ultimate goal. Here, the former problem or behavior will no longer present any temptation or threat. Change is complete, there is no need to make any further effort and this cycle of this change can usually be exited. However, some ex-perts believe that certain problems cannot be terminated but only kept at bay. This is particularly the case where there is any form of addiction – to food, or alcohol, or other addictive substances or behaviors.

Environment for Change

A frequent barrier to success is the environment in which people live. They find a good practitioner, a great practitioner and do some test-ing and get some treatment recommendations, but then they go home to the same life and lifestyle they have been living that got them there in the first place. Usually, making a long lasting change that both reduces, and reverses chronic illness, requires way more than some tests, some hormones, and some supplements. If you are serious, really, really serious about returning your body and mind to a healthful state then there is some "house cleaning" that will have to happen. Making change can be exciting for some, those who thrive on something new, a new start, a new program. For others, change surfaces feelings of fear. Whether you thrive on change or feel terrified by it, try to be kind with yourself as you prepare to change. Here are some common steps that people take to create the environment for a successful return to health.

- Test your hormones and use the BHRT consistently.
- Focus on sleeping – EVERY night.
- Practice adoring yourself more and make self-care a priority.
- Replace high glycemic foods such as pastas and breads with low glycemic foods such as crunchy, tasty, organic vegetables.
- Replace some of the many high stress activities you do with calmer creative hobbies.
- Do more home based activities with kids rather than drive them around endlessly to activities.
- Require kids to do more chores so it is not all on you (provide internet access as an incentive when they help around the house).
- Accept help, trust others to do things you could probably do better.
- Drink water in between a sip of something alcoholic.
- Walk with a friend instead of saying you will do it alone (and then don't).
- Replace negative people in your life with positive supportive people.
- Return to or develop a deeper spiritual connection.

Matrix of Change Choices

In the appendix is a Matrix for Change. The Matrix lists the chapters and has space for you to list the activities related to each of the associated behaviors that are harmful and contribute to your chronic state. The Matrix also has space for you to lists the positive things you are going to do to support your return to health. You can also download the matrix from: www.aforecastforhealth.com.

Remember that the work you choose to do will be in partnership with the treatment recommendations that your practitioner makes.

Remember too, that while your practitioner is using all their skill and knowledge and wisdom to make treatment recommendations, you are the one who chooses to use them and put their ideas to work.

Your Visit with the Practitioner

When you visit your practitioner to begin finding the root cause of your health situation you can expect the following:

1. First patient exam which will include an extensive health history, and may include an analysis of emotional trauma history
2. Physical exam that may include muscle testing to diagnose organ issues
3. Ordering some but not likely all of the following testing:
   - Salivary hormone testing
   - Urinary neurotransmitter testing
   - Blood Panels, including full Thyroid panel
   - Heavy metal testing
   - Food allergy testing
   - Sleep study
   - Genetic tendency testing
   - Micronutrient testing
4. Second visit to review results and receive the practitioners diagnosis
   - Review results of testing
   - Discuss the sequence of treatment approaches
   - Begin treatment

You will be given time, attention, and thoughtful information about a path that you can take to becoming well again. You get to decide how far along that path you want to go and at what pace. Your practitioner is your partner on this path, a resource to help you determine your best health related options and, if all goes well, this partnership with your practitioner could turn out to be a long term relationship. A good practitioner will spend time with you, listening to your health concerns and help you decide on your path back to health and onward into wellness. You can correct long term patterns and rebuild nutritional health, physical health, restful sleep, as well as reduce the state of inflammation in your body. As you continue to age, your natural hormone levels will fluctuate, stresses will sometimes arise, and the rate at which repair happens will slow over time. Your ongoing partnership with your practitioner can be your route to a long, happy, comfortable, pain free, productive life.

Of course – if you like being a victim...

Money and Change

Now for the heavy hitting conversation. When embarking on this work with a practitioner, it is wise to be prepared for the financial cost. There are an increasing number of health insurance plans (in the US) that will provide some funds for preventative wellness and alternative care, however, many of the laboratories that will be providing the testing services will not be covered costs or will be out of network. Depending on your insurance plan, practitioner's fees may also be applied to a deductible. That means you are likely to be paying for the practitioner's services, much of the necessary testing, and also have costs related to treatment solutions.

Why does Integrative Medicine have a cost to it?

Some people may be surprised by the rates that practitioners charge for their services. Consider this – most practitioners will have undertaken at least eight years post high school education to acquire their medical knowledge. In addition, there are requirements for continuing medical education to keep current with the new discoveries in their field. Practitioners, while here to heal, also have to be business people: they have to rent space, pay staff, keep the lights on, pay themselves. Nobody baulks at paying a lawyer their usual high fee for services, or a plumber or house painter, why is it that we hesitate to pay a practitioner a fee for not just their knowledge, but their skill. Here are some common beliefs that people have about paying for healthcare:

- Healthcare is a right – why should I have to pay for it?
- Insurance should cover this, I pay high enough premiums
- Practitioners should do this work because they care, not because they want to make money

As you read that quick list – be honest with yourself about which beliefs you hold, then understand that those are just beliefs, not facts. To work with an Integrative Medicine practitioner you may have to make some tough financial choices, you may need to forgo saving, or reduce spending on some other things in order to invest in your health. It can be an eye opening exercise to list the items that you spend money on that just help you get by and make you feel better, if only for a short time. Common expenses are:

- Expensive designer coffee once a day – $80 a month
- Eating out if too tired to cook –$250 a month
- Alcoholic drinks to help calm you down – $100 a month
- Cigarettes to calm you down – $50 a month
- Junk food on the run instead of healthy snacks – $60 a month
- Sugar and candy and energy drink for energy – $50 a month
- Shopping spree because "I deserve a treat" – $150 a month

The choice is yours to decide just how important is it to feel well and healthy. Whatever your opinions on healthcare and health insurance, one things is certain, there will be some costs that come out of your pocket, so you may as well start to think about the whole subject in a different way; the more resistance you put up about the financial aspect, the more resistant you are likely to be to take action towards change.

Consider for a moment your house or your car or your personal property. You pay an insurance premium that covers serious events like trees falling through the roof, collisions with other cars, or theft of property. Insurance is designed to be there for the unseen and unwanted serious events. Insurance does not pay for home maintenance such as repainting, or replacing old lead piping, nor does it pay for the oil change on your car or replacing the cylinder head gasket – those are all ongoing maintenance costs that you pay for out of your monthly budget or savings. We pay those maintenance costs without real complaint, it is just how it works. So why do we look at health insurance as something different? The actions you take to maintain your body, are just that, repair and maintenance actions. We engage a practitioner to identify and treat long term chronic conditions in the body, in a somewhat similar way as we might engage an electrician to rewire an aging house, or get a service overhaul on the car that replaces needed parts on schedule.

Health insurance does a reasonable job of covering the acute situations, like emergency surgery, treatment for cancer or other serious organ disease. The question is, do you really want to neglect maintenance of your body long enough to get to the point of serious illness just to get insurance to pay for your costs? And anyway, co-pays on a serious illness can be far more expensive in the long run than what you could spend on some upfront body repair and maintenance right now. If you don't repair a leak in the roof when it starts, five years later you could end up with dry rot which causes the entire roof and ceiling to collapse, creating far greater expense and disruption than fixing the original small leak. If you don't invest in repairing your health now, it will cost more down the road, and you will also feel really crappy.

One of the core principles of Integrative Medicine is the belief that prevention is preferable to treatment whenever possible. This approach is almost always safer, more effective, and less expensive. Unfortunately, the U.S. health care system currently does not "incentivize" many aspects of preventive/wellness care. If we are to truly improve health, we must shift towards valuing wellness care and prevention. Until that happens, increasingly people are now allocating a certain amount into their monthly budget for healthcare that is over and above health insurance payments. This is now a reality. As we have explored in the previous chapters, our chosen lifestyles, along with degradations in environmental and food quality, mean the body is up against some serious barriers in terms of maintaining a healthful state. It is wise now to allocate money for health – such as gym membership, good walking shoes, a new bike for cycling to work, organic vegetables, quality supplements, hormone prescriptions, practitioner appointments, annual testing. If you are in the place where you are thinking "this isn't how it should be," perhaps you are right, however, it is how it is.

If you continue to find yourself grumbling about that concept, think about how people save for retirement. While state/federal pension plans will be one source of income for retirement, most people recognize that it is unlikely to be enough to live on. Many people will chose to defer the use of funds today, to save money for use in retirement. Why not apply that principle to your body and your health – invest time and money in your body now, so it is available for full use in the future. I know that I would prefer to live to ninety years or more, thoroughly active, pain free, and able to enjoy all those years.

Relationship and Change

The most profound relationship we have through our life is the one we have with our self. We are the only one who is always there, all the way through our entire life. Yes, we are social animals and we need others to varying degrees for safety, connection, mutual benefit and so on, but really, when you stop and think about it – we are our own constant companion. Wherever we go – there we are. It doesn't matter if we move to a new home, a new city, a new country, what we take with us each time is ourselves. Relationships with others therefore, begin and end with our relationship with our self. To learn to love the self can be a lifetime's work. As multiple research studies have shown, early childhood experiences have a huge impact on our lives and how we then live as adults. It is more common than not that our sweet little selves were not treated well as we grew up. As babies, toddlers, children, teens, we learned so many messages that end up being harmful. It is not the work of this book to describe more details here because there is plenty to read in the popular press about this subject. What is relevant here is that if we grow up with messages of "I am not good" or "I am not worth enough/anything," then valuing the self enough to care for ourselves can be very difficult.

It took me being very ill with ankylosing spondylitis and then finding a medication to manage it, for me to bring myself up straight and begin to really take care of myself. Over time I have developed the practice of sacred selfishness, a term I use to describe my commitment to putting myself first in order to then give to those who need what I can provide. If I am not strong and whole and at peace with myself, I cannot bring my best to others without it depleting me.

Sacred selfishness is not "it is all about me, me, me", it is about making sure I take care of myself first, before anyone else, so that I can give to others from a strong place. Sacred selfishness is also about taking responsibility for the self, refusing to be a victim, and not looking to others to take care of us. When we do look to others to take care of us, we put ourselves back into that child-like state of "mommy, daddy, where are you, take care of me." And yet we are adults, and we need to grow up and take gentle, kind, respectful responsibility for ourselves. If this is hard for you, then it could be worthwhile to explore with a therapist why you find this difficult.

As I stepped into taking care of myself and my needs, I also took responsibility for my own emotions, paying attention frequently to any fear-based reactions. In so doing, I realized it is never appropriate to blame anyone else for how I am feeling. I am responsible for how I feel. I gradually began to notice my physical sensations and to match those sensations with what was going on with my emotions. I began to recognize fear in my body (my gut), hurt (in my hips), affection (my heart), self-silencing (a tightness in my throat) and so on. I began to know when I did not want to do something, even though my initial response was to please and say, "Yes, I will do that". Gradually I began to take care of *my* needs. I made sure I got at least seven hours sleep each night. I found time to swim regularly, I made time for creative expression, I moved away from relationships that no longer nurtured and supported me, I invested in my career, and I committed to my ongoing self learning and spiritual growth.

I am still a work in progress, far, far, far from "perfect" but I now live life from a strong self nurturing place. It is that strong place that allows me to find the courage to write this book and bring this information to you. Just even writing that sentence brings tears to my eyes; tears of gratitude and appreciation for how far I have come on my journey. There are plenty of resources available to help you connect with yourself in a deeper way, counsellors with whom you can talk, or spiritual teachers from whom you can learn. Your healing journey will be faster, smoother, more successful, if you first change your relationship with yourself to one of loving acceptance and nurturance.

Whatever type of healthcare practitioner you choose to work with on your healing journey, remember that he or she is a guide who is practicing the art of diagnosing and treating. The body is not black and white, it is a complex interaction of biochemistry and emotion. No practitioner is a miracle worker, and no practitioner is able to support your healing unless you really want to heal.

If you have found this book to be helpful in anyway, large or small, then it has all been worthwhile. Please pass on the information about the book to people you know who could also take useful information from it and step onto their healing path.

> I wish you luck, I wish you strength,
> I wish you health, and I wish you joy.

> *Yours, in light*
> Kate Wells

APPENDIX

GUIDE TO APPENDICES

The first draft of this book contained far more pages. After kind and thoughtful feedback from several people it has been reduced to this hopefully neat and accessible size, with quick reference information organized into Appendices:

- **Appendix A** In addition to the information in this book there are resources available for further reading. Also listed are some of the journals and articles that provided data and technical information.

- **Appendix B** shows a list of common symptoms associated with hormone imbalance. Hormone balance is a foundational aspect of Integrative Medicine. I encourage you to use this checklist to see what your own picture of hormone balance looks like.

- **Appendix C** is a Matrix for Change to prompt thoughts about what are the next right things for your health.

- **Appendix D** has information on websites and organizations that are resources for you in seeking an Integrative Medicine Practitioner.

- **Appendix E** contains a glossary of words. My intention was to keep language straightforward, but there are plenty of scientific words that might be unfamiliar, these are listed in the glossary.

- **Appendix F** is a Sleep Diary for you to use to collect data prior to working with your practitioner.

- **Appendix G** contains a list of energetic biofeedback device manufacturers.

- **Appendix H** contains a list of testing laboratories.

Appendix A

Brief Bibliography and Extended Reading Options

This book is about the beautiful biochemistry of the human body and the human mind. The books listed below are a fraction of the resources I have read over many years from which I have culled snippets of useful information. I list books that could be good references for extended reading if you want to learn more. Because I started reading long before I knew I would be writing, I decided it would be herculean task to list the hundreds of articles I read and presentations I heard that helped build the content of this particular book. If you come across something specific in the text that you want to know more about, you are welcome to contact me through www.aforecastforhealth.com and I will see if I can dig out a particular reference for you. References are listed in the general order of the chapters.

Books and Articles

Manhattan, B. The Whole systems medicine of tomorrow: a half-century perspective. *Explore*. 2011. Vol 7 No.4

Abrams, D. Integrative Medicine in America. *Global Advances in Health and Medicine*. 2012. Vol 1 No.3

US Burden of Disease Collaborators. The State of US Health, 1990-2010. Burden of Diseases, Injuries, and Risk Factors. *JAMA*. 2013;310(6):591-606

Lloyd, I. The Root Cause of Disease is Never a Symptom. *Vital Link CAND* 2008, Vol 15 Issue 3

Hyman, M. Dangerous Spin Doctors: Seven steps to protect yourself from deception in medical research. *Explore*. 2011 Vol 7, No.2

Champe, P, Harvey, R, Ferrier, D (2005) *Biochemistry 3rd Ed.* Lippincott, Williams & Wilkins.

Lifestyle Medicine - Evidence Review. American College of Preventive Medicine 2009

Medina, J (2008) *Brain Rules: 12 Principles for Surviving and Thriving at Work, Home, and School.* Pear Press

Shallenberger, F (2002). *Bursting With Energy.* InMED Publishing

Bongiorno, P. Depression and Sleep. *NDNR* 2013, Vol 9 Issue 3

Gross, C et al. Mindfulness-based stress reduction versus Pharmacotherapy for Chronic Primary Insomnia: A Randomized Controlled Clinical Trial. *Explore* 2011, Vol 7, No 2

Hogl B, Kiechl S, Willeir, J et al. Restless legs syndrome: a community based-study of prevalaence, severity, and risk factors. *Neurology*, 2005; 64:1920-1924

Waters AS. Toward a better definition of restless legs syndrome. The international

Restless Legs Syndrome Study Group. *Mov Disord* 1995; 10:634-642

Patrick L. Restless Legs Syndrome: Pathophysicology and the role of iron and folate. *Alternative Medicine Review,* Vol 12 No.2 2007

Lewy, A. Circadian misalignment in mood disturbances. *Current Psychiatry Reports.* December 2009, Volume 11, Issue 6, pp 459-465

Buijs RM et al. The biological clock tunes the organs of the body: timing by hormones and the autonomic nervous system. *J Endocrinol* April 1, 2003 177 17-26

Ackerman, J. (2007) *Sex, Sleep, Eat, Drink, Dream; A Day in the Life of Your Body.* First Mariner Books

Diamond, J (1992) *The Third Chimpanzee the Evolution and Future of the Human Animal.* Harper Perennial

Lombardo, G T. (2005) *Sleep to Save Your Life, the Complete Guide to Living Longer and Healthier Through Restorative Sleep.* Collins

Morgan, D. (1996) *Sleep Secrets for Shift Workers & People with Off-Beat Schedules.* Whole Person Associates

Schenck, C.H. (2007) Sleep. *The Mysteries, the Problems, and the Solutions.* Avery

Wiley T.S. with Formby, B. (2000) *Lights Out – Sleep, Sugar, and Survival.* Pocket Books

Pfaffe T, et al. Diagnostic Potential of Saliva: Current State and Future Applications. *Clinical Chemistry* 2011. 57:5 675-687

Mcculloch, F. Supporting the Luteal Phase with integrative medicine. *NDNR* 2012. Vol 8 Issue 8

McEwen B. Estrogen Actions throughout the Brain, *The Endocrine Society,* Vol. 57, No. 1, 2002, pp. 357-384

Coelingh Bennink HJT: Are all estrogens the same? *Maturitas* 47, 2004. 269-275

Goodman M: Are all estrogens created equal? A review of oral vs, transdermal therapy. *Jrnl Women's Health.* Vol 21, No. 2 2012

Frackiewicz EJ, Cutler N: Women's healthcare during the perimenopause. *J AM Pharm Asoc* 40(6): 800-811, 2000

Selby C. Sex hormone binding globulin: origin, function and clinical significance. *Ann Clin Biochem* 1990; 27:532-41

Head K. Estriol: Safety and Efficacy. *Alternative Medicine Review* Vol 3, No. 2, 1998

McEwen B, Biegon, A. Modulation by Estradiol of Serotonin1 receptors in brain. *Journal of Neuroscience* Vol 2 no.2 199-205 1982

Yamada, Y., et al. Changes in serum sex hormone profiles after short-term low-does administration of dehydroepiandostern one (DHEA) to young and elderly persons. *Endocr J* 2007 Feb;54(1):153-62

Fitzpatrick LA, et al. Comparison of regimens containing oral micronized progesterone or medroxyprogesterone acetate on quality of life in postmenopausal women: a cross-sectional survey. *J Women's Health Gender Based Med.* 2000; 9: 381-387.

Murkes D, et al. Effects of percutaneous estradiol-oral progesterone versus oral conjugated equine estrogens-medroxyprogesterone acetate on breast cell proliferation and bcl-2 protein in healthy women. *Fertil Steril.* 2011; 95: 1188-91.

Bernstein P, Pohost G. Progesterone, progestins and the heart. *Rev Cardiovasc Med.* 2010; 11: 228-36.

Rabijewski, M and Zgliczynski, W "Positive effects of DHEA therapy on insulin resistance and lipids in men with angiographically verified coronary heart disease – preliminary study" *Endokrynol* Pol. 2005 Nov-Dec; 56(6):904-10

Suhr J et el. The relation of salivary cortisol to patterns of performance on a word list learning task in healthy older adults. *Psychoneuroendocrinology* Volume 33, Issue 9, October 2008, Pages 1293–1296

Lee, J Hanley, J, Hopkins V. (1999). *What Your Doctor May Not Tel You About Postmenopause.* Wellness Central

Lee, J Hanley, J, Hopkins V. (1999). *What Your Doctor May Not Tel You About Premenopause.* Wellness Central

Lommen, E.T & Mead J.H. (2012) *Slim, Sane and Sexy.* Calaroga Publishing

Sichel, D & Driscoll J,(1999). *Women's Moods : What Every Woman Must Know About Hormones, the Brain, and Emotional Health.* New York

WHI. Risks and benefits of estrogen plus progestin in healthy postmenopausal women. Principal results from the women's health initiative randomized controlled trial. *JAMA.* 2002;288(3):321-333

Crinnion, W. Why it is best to avoid farmed salmon. *Vital Link CAND* 2008 Vol 15, Issue 2

Nash, G Food Sensitivities and Epigenetics, *NDNR,* 2013, Vol 9 Issue 4

DeBusk, R, Sierpina, V, Kreitzer, MJ. Applying Functional Nutrition for chronic disease prevention and management: bridging nutrition and functional medicine in 21st century healthcare. *Explore,* 2011 Vol 7, No.1

Metcalfe, D. Genetically Modified Foods, Mini-monograph. *Environmental Health Perspectives.* 2003. Vol 111, No.8

Gaby, A: The role of hidden food allergy/intolerance in chronic disease. *Alternative Medicine Review,* Vol 3 No. 2 1998

Robeva R et. Al, Melatonin–insulin interactions in patients with metabolic syndrome. *Jn Pineal Research.* Volume 44, Issue 1, pages 52–56, January 2008

Braly, J. (2000) *Food Allergy Relief.* Keats Publishing

Fields, D (2009) *The Other Brain.* Simon and Schuster

Guilliams, T.G (2014) *Supplementing Dietary Nutrients, A Guide for Healthcare Professionals.* Point Institute

Head, K. (2000). *Everything You Need to Know About Diabetes.* Prima Health

Rubin, J & Brasco J, (2003) *Restoring Your Digestive Health.* Kensington

Vojdani, A. For the Assessment of Intestinal Permeability, Size Matters. *Alt Therapies,* 2013, Vol 19. No.1

Bradley R et al. Adjunctive Naturopathic care for type 2 diabetes: patient reported and clinical outcomes after 1 year. *Integrative Medicine* 2012. Vol 11 No. 6

Besedovsky HO, del ReyA: The cytokine-HPA axis feedback circuit. Z

Rheumatology 59 (Suppl 2): 11/26-11/30, 2000

Byers M, Bonica J. *Peripheral pain mechanisms and nonciceptor plasticity. Bonica's Management of Pain 3rd ed.* Lippincott Williams & Wilkins, 2001, pp26-72

Epel Elissa. *Psychological and metabolic stress: a recipe for accelerated cellular aging?* University of CA, Department of Psychiatry, San Francisco, CA

Bonakdar, R. Obesity-related pain: time for a new approach that target systemic inflammation. *Chronic Pain Perspectives* 2013; 62(9): s22-s28

Brain Facts, A primer on the brain and nervous system. Society for Neuroscience. 2005

Rosas-Ballina, Tracey, KJ: Cholinergic control of inflammation. *Journal of Internal Medicine.* 265; 663-679 2009

Blalock JE, The immune system as a sensory organ. *J Immunology* 1984; 132: 126-38

Clauw, D : Targeting neurotransmitters: modulating pain response. *Johns Hopkins Advanced Studies in Medicine Proceedings* Vol 9 Nov 2009

Aloisi AM, Bonifazi M: Sex hormones, central nervous system and pain. *Hormones and Behavior* 50 (2006) 1-7

Meletis C, Berzow R: Brain Pain: the role for neuromodulation and novel applications of humulus lupulus. *Townsend Letter* October 2012

Juhl J: Fibromyalgia and the Serotonin pathway. *Alternative Medicine Review.* Vol 3 No. 5 1998

Elgha E et al. Cognitive Dysfunction, Hippocampal Atrophy and Glucocorticoid Feedback in Alzheimer's Disease, *Biological Psychiatry,* Volume 59, Issue 2, 15 January 2006, Pages 155–161

Cutolo M et al. Circadian rhythms in RA. *Ann Rheum Dis* 2003;62:593-596

Amen, D.G. (2002) *Healing the Hardware of the Soul.* Free Press

Amen, DG (2005) *Making a Good Brain Great.* Harmony Books

Ashcroft. F (2012) .*The Spark of Life – Electricity in the Human Body.* WW Norton & Company

Barnard, N (1998). *Foods That Fight Pain.* New York. Three Rivers Press

Becker, R.O, Selden, G (1985). *The Body Electric, Electromagnetism and the Foundation of Life.* William Morrow

Breedove S.M. (2010) *Biological Psychology: An Introduction to Behavioral, Cognitive and Clinical Neuroscience 6th Ed.* Sinauer Associates

Blatman, Hal (2002/2006) *The Art of Body Maintenance: Winners Guide to Pain Relief.* Danua Press LLC

Gibney, M.J. (1986). *Nutrition Diet and Health.* Cambridge University Press

Jawer, M.A with Micozzi, M.S. (2009) *Spiritual Anatomy of Emotion How Feelings Link the Brain, the Body and the Sixth Sense.* Park Street Press

Kirsch, I (2009) *The Emperor's New Drugs Exploding the Antidepressant Myth.* Random House

Oschman, J (2000). *Energy Medicine, The Scientific Basis.* Elsevier Limited

Sobel,D. Klein A, (1989) *Arthritis, What Really Works.* Robinson Publishing

Stanton, H.E. (1981). *The Healing Factor.* Macdonald Optima

Young, M (2002) *Women and Pain, Why It Hurts and What You Can Do.* Hyperion

Warburton, DER, Nicol, CW, Bredin SSD. Health benefits of physical activity: the evidence. *CMAJ* March 14, 2006. 174(6) 801-809

Crowley, C Lodge, H.S (2004,2005) *Younger Next Year for Women.* Workman Publishing Company

Friel, J (2006). *Total Heart Rate Training.* Ulysses Press

Morehouse, L Gross, L (1977) *Total Fitness in 30 Minutes a Week.* Grafton

Mercury Exposure Issue. *Vital Link CAND* 2010 Vol 17, Issue 1

Burnett, K. Genius, S: Chronic Illness and Toxic Exposure. *Integrative Medicine* 2013. Vol 12, No.3

Khan SJ, Muafia,S, Nasreen, Z, Salariya AM. Genetically Modified Organisms: Food security or threat to food safety. *Pakistan Journal of Science* 2012. Vol 64 No.2

Taylor, J (1988) *The Complete Guide to Mercury Toxicity from Dental Fillings.* Scripps Publishing

Beck, D. Life balance. Listening to our bodies to achieve work-life balance. *NDNR* 2012 Vol 8 Issue 6

Begley, Sharron. I Can't Think. *Nature.* 2011, March 7

Chapman, CR, Tuckett, RP Song CW. Pain and stress in s systems perspective: reciprocal neural, endocrine, and immune interactions. *J Pain.* 2008 Feb;9(2):122-45

Berridge CW, Waterhouse BD. The locus coeruleus-nor-adrenergic system: modulation of behavioral state and state-dependent cognitive processes. *Brain Res Rev* 42:33-84 2003

Chrousos GP, Gold PW: A healthy body in a healthy mind- and vice versa - the damaging power of "uncontrollable" stress. *J Clin Endocrinology Metab* 1998; 83: 1842-1845

Doidge, N (2007) *The Brian that changes Itself, Stories of Personal Triumph from the Frontiers of Brain Science.* Penguin

Wilson, J (2001) *Adrenal Fatigue. The 21st Century Stress Syndrome.* Smart Publications

APPENDIX B
Health Check, Women's Symptom Review

Symptom	none	mild	moderate	severe
Difficulty Concentrating				
Increased Forgetfulness				
Foggy Thinking				
Tearful				
Depressed				
Mood Swings				
Fluid Retention / Bloating				
Cold Extremities				
Stress				
Anxious				
Irritable				
Nervous				
Decreased Mental Sharpness				
Morning Fatigue				
Afternoon Fatigue				
Evening Fatigue				
Excessive Worry				
Difficulty Falling Asleep				
Difficulty Staying Asleep				
Decreased Stamina				
Diminished Motivation				
Fibromyalgia				
Ringing in Ears				
Allergies				
Headaches/Migraines				
Dizzy Spells				
Sugar Cravings				
Addictive Behavior				
Poor Impulse Control				
Obsessive Behavior (OCD)				
Craving Food, Alcohol, Tobacco or Other				
Constipation				
Goiter				
Cold Body Temperature				
Hoarseness				

Symptom	none	mild	moderate	severe
Hair Dry or Brittle				
Nails Breaking or Brittle				
Slow Pulse Rate				
Rapid Heartbeat				
Heart Fluttering/Palpitations				
Incontinence				
Hot Flashes				
Night Sweats				
Infertility Problems				
Acne				
Scalp Hair Loss				
Weight Gain-Hips				
Weight Gain-Waist				
High Cholesterol				
Elevated Triglycerides				
Decreased Libido				
Decreased Muscle Size				
Decreased Flexibility				
Burned Out Feeling				
Sore Muscles				
Increased Joint Pain				
Neck or Back Pain				
Bone Loss				
Thinning Skin				
Rapid Aging				
Aches and Pains				
IBS				
Vaginal Dryness				
Irregular Periods				
Uterine Fibroids				
Tender Breasts				
Fibrocystic Breasts				
Increased Facial / Body Hair				
Vaginal Dryness				

Printed with permission from Labrix Clinical Services

Appendix C
Matrix For Change
My plan of action for self-care and making the most of my potential

Chapter	My current actions that could use some redirection	Changes I will make to nurture myself	*When* I will add more self care	*Why* I will add more self care
Sleep				
Hormones				
Nutrition				
Pain				
Exercise				
Toxicity				
Stress				

APPENDIX D
Find A Practitioner

There are plenty of organizations and companies that can help you find a practitioner to work with in your area. Some resources are listed below. For additional resources as I find them, check out the website at www.aforecastforhealth.com

www.functionalmedicine.org/practitioner_search.aspx?id=117

www.labrix.com/FindPractitioner

www.spectracell.com/patients/get-tested/

www.naturopathic.org/AF_MemberDirectory.asp?version=2

acam.site-ym.com/search/custom.asp?id=1758

www.councildid.com/10230/index.html

www.icimed.com/member_search.php

www.wellness.com/find/integrative%20doctor

my.clevelandclinic.org/services/wellness/integrative-medicine/treatments-services

www.xymogen.com/patients/find-practitioner.aspx

Glossary Of Terms

Acetylcholine   A short-acting neurotransmitter, widely distributed in the body, that functions as a nervous system stimulant, a vasodilator, and a cardiac depressant.

Adrenal dysfunction   Adrenal dysfunction is a collection of signs and symptoms, known as a syndrome, that results when the adrenal glands function below the necessary level.

Adrenal gland   A small gland located on top of the kidney. The adrenal glands produce hormones that help control heart rate, blood pressure, the way the body uses food, the levels of minerals such as sodium and potassium in the blood, and other functions particularly involved in stress reactions.

Adrenal medulla   The inner, reddish-brown portion of the adrenal gland that synthesizes, stores, and releases epinephrine and norepinephrine.

Adrenarche   An increase in the production of androgens by the adrenal cortex that usually occurs during the eighth or ninth year of life.

Aldosterone   A corticosteroid hormone that stimulates absorption of sodium by the kidneys and so regulates water and salt balance.

Allopathic   Relating to or being a system of medicine that aims to combat disease by using remedies (as drugs or surgery) which produce effects that are different from or incompatible with those of the disease being treated.

Amino acid   An amino acid is a type of organic acid that contains an acid functional group and an amine functional group on adjacent carbon atoms. Amino acids are considered to be the building blocks of proteins.

Anabolic hormone   An anabolic hormone is a chemical that encourages cellular growth, usually building molecules up and into something new once they have been broken down.

Androsteindione   A steroid produced in the adrenal gland that is a precursor to testosterone and other male hormones (androgens).

Anovulation   Anovulation is a condition in which the ovary does not release a ripened egg each month as part of a woman's normal cycle in her reproductive years.

Antibody   An antibody is a protein molecule that can be found in the blood and is intended to attack bacteria, viruses, and transplanted organs.

Antigens   An antigen is a harmful substance which enters the body and causes the body to make antibodies as a response.

Antioxidant   A chemical substance that prevents or slows down the damage that oxygen (free radicals) does to organisms or to food.

Apoptosis A form of cell death in which a programmed sequence of events leads to the elimination of cells without releasing harmful substances into the surrounding area.

Autoimmune disease A disease in which the body produces antibodies that attack its own tissues, leading to the deterioration and in some cases to the destruction of such tissue.

Autonomic nervous system The definition of an autonomic nervous system is the bodily process that controls all involuntary actions such as breathing and digestion.

BHRT Bioidentical Hormone Replacement Therapy

Bile A bitter greenish-brown alkaline fluid that aids digestion and is secreted by the liver and stored in the gallbladder.

Binding globulins Blood proteins that bind to different types of hormones.

Blood-brain barrier A filtering mechanism of the capillaries that carry blood to the brain and spinal cord tissue, blocking the passage of certain substances.

Carbohydrate An organic compound that occurs in living tissues or food and that can be broken down into energy by humans or animals.

Cell differentiation The process by which a cell becomes specialized in order to perform a specific function, as in the case of a liver cell, a blood cell, or a neuron.

Cellular waste Cellular waste products are formed as a by-product of cellular respiration, a series of processes and reactions that generate energy for the cell.

Circadian rhythm disorders The natural sleep-wake rhythm is known as the circadian rhythm. A disruption of this rhythm may be considered a circadian rhythm sleep disorder.

Collagen The fibrous protein constituent of bone, cartilage, tendon, and other connective tissue.

Conjugate A compound formed by the joining of two or more chemical compounds.

Corpus luteum A yellow, progesterone-secreting mass of cells that forms from an ovarian follicle after the release of a mature egg.

Corticotrophin-releasing hormone Corticotropin-releasing hormone (CRH) also known as corticotropin-releasing factor (CRF) is a peptide hormone and neurotransmitter involved in the stress response.

Cortisol Cortisol is a steroid hormone produced in the adrenal gland that is required for normal endocrine function.

Cortisol awakening response The cortisol awakening response is an increase of about 50% in cortisol levels occurring 30 minutes after awakening in the morning in most people.

Cytochrome p450s A group of enzymes involved in drug metabolism and found in high levels in the liver.

Cytokines Cytokines are cell signaling molecules that aid cell to cell communication in immune responses and stimulate the movement of cells towards sites of inflammation, infection and trauma.

Delayed sleep phase disorder Delayed sleep phase is an internal sleep clock (circadian rhythm) sleep disorder in which your sleep pattern is delayed two hours or more from a normal sleep.

DHEA Dehydroepiandrosterone is an androgenic steroid hormone secreted mainly in the adrenal gland. DHEA is the biologically active form which can be converted into androgens and estrogen and only DHEA (not DHEAS) is protective for the brain.

DHEA(s) Sulphated DHEA (DHEAS). DHEAS is the inactive stored reservoir form of DHEA. DHEAS levels do not reflect biologically active DHEA levels.

Dopamine Dopamine is a type of neurotransmitter that is important for a number of different functions in the brain.

Dysbiosis Dysbiosis refers to microbial imbalance on or inside the body. Dysbiosis is most commonly reported as a condition in the digestive tract.

Endocrine system The endocrine system refers to the collection of glands of an organism that secrete hormones directly into the circulatory system to be carried towards a distant target organ.

Endometrium The mucous membrane lining of the uterus (womb).

Endorphin A hormonal compound that is made by the body in response to pain or extreme physical exertion that affect receptors in the brain, often reducing the sensation of pain or stress.

Endothelium The endothelium is the thin layer of simple cells that lines the interior surface of blood vessels and lymphatic vessels.

Endotoxin lps A toxin that forms an integral part of the cell wall of certain bacteria and is only released upon destruction of the bacterial cell.

Enzyme Any protein that acts as a catalyst, increasing the rate at which a chemical reaction occurs. The human body probably contains about 10,000 different enzymes.

Epinephrine A hormone and a neurotransmitter produced primarily by the adrenal glands in response to stress; called also adrenaline.

Estradiol A major estrogen hormone produced by the ovaries.

Estriol An estrogen that is a metabolite of estradiol and is the main estrogen secreted by the placenta during pregnancy.

Estrone A naturally occurring weak estrogenic hormone secreted by the ovaries, often the most common estrogen in post menopausal women.

Fasting glucose test A check of a person's blood glucose level after the person has not eaten for 8 to 12 hours (usually overnight).

Fibrinogen A plasma protein that is produced in the liver and is converted into fibrin during blood clot formation.

Fibroid A common benign tumor of the uterus.

Follicle In the female reproductive system, a follicle is a fluid-filled sac that contains an immature egg, or oocyte. Follicles are found in the ovaries.

Free radicals An atom or group of atoms that has at least one unpaired electron and is therefore unstable and highly reactive.

GABA Gamma-aminobutyric acid: a biologically active substance found in plants and in brain and other animal tissues; it is a neurotransmitter that inhibits (calms) activation of neurons.

Genetic variant A variation in the normal structure of a gene.

Ghrelin A hormone that stimulates the feeling of hunger.

Glucose A simple sugar that is an important energy source in living organisms and is a component of many carbohydrates.

Glucose tolerance test A test of the body's ability to metabolize glucose that involves the administration of a measured dose of glucose to the fasting stomach and the determination of glucose levels in the blood and urine at measured intervals thereafter.

Glutamate Glutamate is an amino acid that acts as a neurotransmitter. Glutamate sends chemical messages in the brain by "exciting" neurons that are sensitive to it.

Glycogen The stored form of glucose, made up of many connected glucose molecules.

Glucagon A hormone produced by the pancreas that stimulates an increase in blood sugar levels, thus opposing the action of insulin.

High density lipoprotein A lipoprotein (fat and protein combination molecule) that removes cholesterol from the blood and is associated with a reduced risk of atherosclerosis and heart disease.

Histamine A compound that is released by cells in response to injury and in allergic and inflammatory reactions, causing contraction of smooth muscle and dilation of capillaries.

Homeostasis A property of cells, tissues, and organisms that allows the maintenance and regulation of the stability and constancy needed to function properly.

Hormone A regulatory substance produced in one place and transported in tissue fluids to stimulate specific cells or tissues into action.

HRT Hormone Replacement Therapy.

Hypersomnia Hypersomnia is a condition that causes a person to feel sleepy throughout the day.

Hypertension Abnormally high blood pressure.

Hypocortisolism A state of persistently high levels of circulating cortisol.

Hypothalamus A region of the forebrain below the thalamus that coordinates both the autonomic nervous system and the activity of the pituitary, controlling body temperature, thirst, hunger, and other homeostatic systems, and involved in sleep and emotional activity.

Immune system The integrated body system of organs, tissues, cells, and cell products such as antibodies that differentiates self from nonself and neutralizes potentially pathogenic organisms or substances.

Immunoglobulin antibodies An antibody (AB), also known as an immunoglobulin (Ig), is a protein produced by plasma cells that is used by the immune system to identify and neutralize foreign objects such as bacteria and viruses.

Insulin A hormone produced in the pancreas by the islets of Langerhans that regulates the amount of glucose in the blood.

Integrative medicine Integrative medicine is healing-oriented medicine that takes account of the whole person (body, mind, and spirit), including all aspects of lifestyle. It emphasizes the therapeutic relationship and makes use of all appropriate therapies, both conventional and alternative.

Killer cells A white blood cell (a type of lymphocyte) that destroys infected or cancerous cells.

Lactose Lactose is a sugar derived from galactose and glucose that is found in milk.

Leptin A peptide hormone that is produced by fat cells and plays a role in body weight regulation by acting on the hypothalamus to suppress appetite and burn fat stored in adipose tissue.

Lipase An enzyme from the pancreas that catalyzes the breakdown of fats to fatty acids and glycerol or other alcohols.

Low density lipoprotein A lipoprotein (fat and protein combination molecule) that transports cholesterol from the liver to the tissues of the body.

Luteal phase The luteal phase is the latter phase of the menstrual cycle.

Luteal phase defect A disruption to the normal pattern for the luteal phase.

Luteinizing hormone A hormone secreted by the anterior pituitary gland that stimulates ovulation in females.

Lymph A clear, watery, sometimes faintly yellowish fluid derived from body tissues that contains white blood cells and circulates throughout the lymphatic system. Lymph acts to remove bacteria and certain proteins from the tissues, transport fat from the small intestine, and supply mature lymphocytes to the blood.

Lymphatic system The network of vessels through which lymph drains from the tissues into the blood.

Macrophages A type of white blood cell that ingests foreign material. Macrophages are key players in the immune response to foreign invaders of the body, such as infectious microorganisms. They are normally found in the liver, spleen, and connective tissues of the body.

Mast cells Mast cells are "master regulators" of the immune system. They come from bone marrow and go into all tissues of the body. Mast cells play an important protective role and have been observed as being intimately involved in wound healing and defense against pathogens.

Melatonin A hormone secreted by the pineal gland involved in regulating the sleeping and waking cycles, among other processes.

Menopause Menopause is defined as occurring 12 months after a woman's last menstrual period and marks the end of menstrual cycles.

Metabolic syndrome A cluster of biochemical and physiological abnormalities associated with the development of cardiovascular disease and Type 2 Diabetes.

Metabolism The chemical processes that occur within a living organism in order to maintain life.

Micronutrients An essential nutrient, as a trace mineral or vitamin, that is required by an organism in minute amounts.

Mitochondria Mitochondria are known as the powerhouses of the cell. They are organelles that act like a digestive system which takes in nutrients, breaks them down, and creates energy rich molecules for the cell.

Monooxygenases Any of a group of enzymes that catalyze both the addition of a single oxygen atom from molecular oxygen into a substrate, and the reduction of a second oxygen atom in the substrate to water.

Mutation The changing of the structure of a gene, resulting in a variant form that may be transmitted to subsequent generations.

Nerve growth factor Nerve growth factor (NGF) is a small secreted protein that is important for the growth, maintenance, and survival of certain target neurons (nerve cells). It also functions as a signaling molecule.

Nervous system The network of nerve cells and fibers that transmits nerve impulses between parts of the body.

Neuron A specialized cell transmitting nerve impulses; a nerve cell.

Neuropeptide Neuropeptides are small protein-like molecules (peptides) used by neurons to communicate with each other. They are neuronal signaling molecules that influence the activity of the brain in specific ways.

Nephron The functional unit of the kidney, in which waste products are filtered from the blood, and urine is produced.

Neurotransmitter (including inhibitory and excitatory) A chemical substance, such as acetylcholine or dopamine, which transmits nerve impulses across a synapse.

Neutrophils A type of white blood cell.

Nociceptor A receptor for pain caused by injury, physical or chemical, to body tissues.

Non rem sleep NREM (non-rapid eye movement) sleep is dreamless sleep. During NREM, the brain waves on the electroencephalographic (EEG) recording are typically slow and of high voltage, the breathing and heart rate are slow and regular, the blood pressure is low, and the sleeper is relatively still.

Norepinephrine A hormone and a neurotransmitter produced primarily by the adrenal glands in response to stress; called also nor-adrenaline.

Oophorectomy Surgical removal of one or both ovaries.

Organic acids An organic acid is an organic compound with acidic properties.

Osteoblasts A cell that makes bone. It does so by producing a matrix that then becomes mineralized.

Oxidation Oxidation is the process when oxygen combines with an element, changing the appearance of the element.

Oxidative damage/stress Oxidative stress is essentially an imbalance between the production of free radicals and the ability of the body to counteract or detoxify their harmful effects through neutralization by antioxidants.

Pancreas A large gland behind the stomach that secretes digestive enzymes into the duodenum. Embedded in the pancreas are the islets of Langerhans, which secrete the hormones insulin and glucagon.

Parasympathetic nervous system The part of the involuntary nervous system that serves to slow the heart rate, increase intestinal and glandular activity, and relax the sphincter muscles.

Perimenopause The period of a woman's life before menopause, this can be up to 10 years.

Pituitary gland The major endocrine gland. A pea-sized body attached to the base of the brain, the pituitary is important in controlling growth and development and the functioning of the other endocrine glands.

Polycystic ovarian syndrome Polycystic ovary syndrome is a condition in which a woman has an imbalance of female sex hormones. This may lead to changes in the menstrual cycle, cysts in the ovaries, trouble getting pregnant, and other health problems.

Polymorphism The occurrence of a number of alternative forms within a section of a nucleic acid or protein molecule.

Precursor A substance from which another is formed, especially by metabolic reaction.

Probiotic Live microorganisms that, when administered in adequate amounts, provide a health benefit to the host.

Progesterone A steroid hormone released by the corpus luteum that stimulates the uterus to prepare for pregnancy.

Progestin Synthetic substance that mimics some of the actions of progesterone but does not exactly match the chemical structure of progesterone.

Pro-inflammatory cytokines A proinflammatory cytokine is a cytokine which promotes systemic inflammation.

Prolactin A hormone secreted by the pituitary gland that stimulates lactation (milk production). It also has many other functions, including essential roles in the maintenance of the immune system and appetite modulation.

Prostaglandins One of a number of hormone-like substances that participate in a wide range of body functions such as the contraction and relaxation of smooth muscle, the dilation and constriction of blood vessels, control of blood pressure, and modulation of inflammation.

Protein Proteins are large biological molecules, or macromolecules, consisting of one or more long chains of amino acid residues.

Receptor A region of tissue, or a molecule in a cell membrane, that responds specifically to a particular neurotransmitter, hormone, antigen, or other substance.

REM sleep A stage in the normal sleep cycle during which dreams occur and the body undergoes various physiological changes, including rapid eye movement, loss of reflexes, and increased pulse rate and brain activity.

Serotonin Serotonin is a chemical created by the human body that works as a neurotransmitter.

Sex hormone binding globulin A family of plasma proteins whose function is to bind free sex hormone molecules and thus reduce their function.

Sublingual Under the tongue.

Sucrose A crystalline sugar found in many plants, especially sugar cane, sugar beets, and sugar maple. It is used widely as a sweetener.

Suprachiasmatic nucleus The suprachiasmatic nucleus (SCN) is a tiny region located in the hypothalamus responsible for controlling circadian rhythms.

Synthetic hormones A synthetic substance that acts like a hormone.

T cells A type of white blood cell that is of key importance to the immune system and is at the core of adaptive immunity.

Testosterone A steroid hormone that stimulates development of male secondary sexual characteristics, produced mainly in the testes, but also in the ovaries and adrenal gland.

Thyroid binding globulin A plasma protein whose function is to bind free thyroid hormone molecules and thus reduce their function.

Toxicant A toxicant is any toxic substance.

Toxins Toxicants produced naturally by a living organism.

Trans fats Trans fatty acids are manufactured fats created during a process called hydrogenation, which is aimed at stabilizing polyunsaturated oils to prevent them from becoming rancid and to keep them solid at room temperature.

Triglycerides A triglyceride consists of three molecules of fatty acid combined with a molecule of the alcohol glycerol.

Vasoconstriction The constriction of blood vessels, which increases blood pressure.

Vasomotor Causing or regulating dilation or constriction of the blood vessels.

Villi Microscopic finger-like projections that line the inner wall of the small intestine.

White cells One of the groups of cells the body makes to help fight infections.

Xenobiotics A chemical compound (as a drug, pesticide, or carcinogen) that is foreign to a living organism.

Xenoestrogens Xenoestrogens are synthetic chemicals that mimic or interfere with estrogen in our bodies. They form a subset of a broader group of chemicals known as endocrine disruptors.

Sleep Diary

Fill out this sleep journal every morning for two weeks. It can help you see what gets in the way of a good night's sleep. It could also help your doctor know more about what affects your sleep.

	Day 1	Day 2	Day 3	Day 4	Day 5	Day 6	Day 7
Did you have any caffeinated drinks today?							
Did you have any alcohol within 2–3 hours of bedtime?							
Did you have a heavy meal within 2–3 hours of bedtime?							
What were you doing about one hour before bedtime? (e.g., watching TV)							
What time did you go to bed last night?							
How long did it take you to fall asleep?							
How many times did you wake up during the night?							
How many hours did you sleep last night?							
What time did you wake up this morning?							
How do you feel this morning after waking up?	□ Refreshed □ Somewhat refreshed □ Tired	□ Refreshed □ Somewhat refreshed □ Tired	□ Refreshed □ Somewhat refreshed □ Tired	□ Refreshed □ Somewhat refreshed □ Tired	□ Refreshed □ Somewhat refreshed □ Tired	□ Refreshed □ Somewhat refreshed □ Tired	□ Refreshed □ Somewhat refreshed □ Tired
What may have affected your sleep? (stress, snoring, temperature, physical discomfort)							

APPENDIX G
Information on Bioenergetic Feedback Devices

www.energetic-devices.com/index.html

Manufacturers:

1. Personal Therapy Device
2. e-Lybra 9
3. NES Pro
4. EPFX SCIO QXCI
5. SCENAR
6. ACUSCEN PRO +

APPENDIX H
List of Specialty Testing Labs

All testing laboratories listed here work directly with practitioners of Integrative Medicine. Many of the labs can help you find a practitioner if you are not able to access this testing through your current health care provider.

Name of Laboratory	Type of Testing Offered
Labrix Clinical Services is a specialist laboratory focusing on hormones and neurotransmitters for optimizing neuroendocrine functioning.	Saliva Hormone Testing Saliva Adrenal Function Testing Urine Neurotransmitter Testing
SpectraCell Laboratories, Inc. specialized offerings include the most advanced tests for assessment of nutritional deficiencies and cardiovascular risk.	Micronutrient Testing Cardiovascular Panel
Great Plains Laboratory Inc. is a world leader in providing testing for nutritional factors in chronic illnesses such as autism, fibromyalgia, and AD(H)D.	Organic Acid Testing Heavy Metals Testing
Doctors Data is a specialist and pioneer in essential and toxic elemental testing.	Heavy Metals Testing Immunology and Allergy Testing Microbiology Testing (Gut Health)
US Biotek provides a variety of immunology and chemistry profiles.	Food Allergy Testing Environmental Pollutants Testing Candida Testing
Cyrex Labs is a high-complexity clinical laboratory offering innovative tests designed to detect and monitor autoimmune reactivity's and their possible triggers.	Autoimmunity Screening Food Sensitivity Testing
RealTime Laboratories, Inc. is a clinical laboratory, specializing in the detection of mycotoxins (the toxins produced by molds) in the human body.	Mold and Mycotoxin Testing

Appendix I
Compounding Pharmacy

Many prescriptions written today are for drugs that are made by a company in a manufacturing plant or factory. When you go to the pharmacy, the pharmacist and the pharmacy technicians will fill a prescription from bottles of supplies in the store. Sometimes though, manufactured medications do not meet the needs of some patients. Examples of these situations include:

- A child needs a medication in a liquid form, but it only comes as a capsule.
- A patient needs a medication that is no longer manufactured.
- A patient needs a dose that is not manufactured.
- The commercially available product is not available.
- A patient is allergic or cannot tolerate an ingredient in a manufactured product.

In these and other situations, it will be necessary to make a personalized prescription specifically for one patient. Compounding is the art and science of creating personalized medications.

Compounded medications are "made from scratch" – individual ingredients are mixed together in the exact strength and dosage form required by the patient. This method allows the compounding pharmacist to work with the patient and the prescriber to customize a medication to meet the patient's specific needs.

It used to be that pharmacists compounded just about all prescriptions, and then, starting in the 1950's and 1960's, drug companies started mass producing medications. As more medications were mass produced, the art of compounding began to decline. This left a gap however, because plenty of people need prescription solutions that did not fit the one-size-fits-all model.

Fortunately, compounding has experienced a resurgence as modern technology and innovative techniques and research have allowed more pharmacists to customize medications to meet specific patient needs. Trained, pharmacists can now personalize medicine for patients who need specific medication solutions. Compounding pharmacists are a great resource for both patients and practitioners because they know a lot about how various chemicals used in medications and supplements work both together, and against each other. Some compounding pharmacists have done additional training and can consult with patients directly on health related concerns.

To learn more about Compounding Pharmacy you can visit these websites:

www.iacprx.org

www.pccarx.com

CPSIA information can be obtained
at www.ICGtesting.com
Printed in the USA
FSOW02n1739071015
11960FS

9 780996 297912